Praise for Nourish and Flourish

"Dr. Hans-Thomas Richter is an outstanding scientist who has made a significant contribution to the field of regenerative medicine. His book on the topic of Omega-3 is highly regarded and praised by the medical and academic community, such as the AASCP. His research is highly accurate and informative and can be used to improve the quality of life of people all over the world. His research can be used to develop treatments for various illnesses and diseases. Dr. Richter is highly respected, and his work is invaluable in the field of regenerative medicine. His contribution to the field is truly remarkable, and his work should be highly appreciated and appraised."

—A.J. Farshchian MD, Director to Heal the Earth Foundation, Medical Director for The Center for Regenerative Medicine, Team physician USA Olympic team, Director to The American Academy of Stem Cell Physicians.

"I've dedicated my career to exploring the frontiers of health and wellness, and the Omega-3 revolution is a remarkable addition to this journey. This book masterfully unravels the complex science of Omega-3 fatty acids, shedding light on our common deficiencies and their far-reaching consequences. It's a must-read for anyone seeking to understand the intricate dance of nutrients within our bodies. The author's deep dive into the world of Omega-3 is both enlightening and empowering, providing readers with the knowledge they need to take control of their health. I highly recommend this book to anyone on a quest for a healthier, more vibrant life."

—Dr. Elliot Spencer, Ph.D., Owner at Utah Cord Bank

"The Omega-3 Revolution' is a game-changer in the realm of health and wellness literature. It masterfully unravels the profound impact of Omega-3 fatty acids on our health, particularly their role in aging. The book illuminates how these essential fats can help in preventing the shortening of chromosomes as we age, a revelation that could redefine our approach to longevity and vitality. A must-read for anyone seeking to understand the science of aging and how to navigate it gracefully. This book is not just informative, but transformative!"

Nourish & Flourish

The Fat that Fuels Us:
Omega-3

For my proud son LUKAS
Enjoy your life!
Papa

Hans-Thomas Richter, Ph.D., MAcOM

Nourish & Flourish: The Fat that Fuels Us: Omega-3

First edition, published 2023

By Hans-Thomas Richter, Ph.D.

Cover art by Reprospace.com and Midjourney.com

Paperback ISBN-13: 978-1-952685-73-6

The information provided in this book is designed to provide helpful information on the subjects discussed. This book is not meant to be used, nor should it be used, to diagnose or treat any medical condition. For diagnosis or treatment of any medical problem, consult your own physician. The publisher and author are not responsible for any specific health or allergy needs that may require medical supervision and are not liable for any damages or negative consequences from any treatment, action, application or preparation, to any person reading or following the information in this book. References are provided for informational purposes only and do not constitute endorsement of any websites or other sources.

Please note that the references to Huckleberry Finn and related narratives within this book are purely fictional and used for illustrative purposes only. They do not represent factual accounts or historical events.

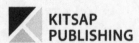

KITSAP PUBLISHING

Published by Kitsap Publishing
Poulsbo, WA 98370
www.KitsapPublishing.com

Contents

Dedication

To my spouse, my rock, who has journeyed with me through every high and low. To my children, who inspire me every day to learn more, do more, and be more.

This book is lovingly dedicated to my entire family - the roots from which I've grown and the branches that continue to expand. To my parents, who nurtured me with love and instilled in me the value of knowledge. To my siblings, whose companionship and support have been my constant. And to my extended family, whose diverse stories and experiences have enriched my own. Each one of you has played a part in shaping who I am today, and for that, I am eternally grateful. This book is a testament to our shared love, resilience, and pursuit of knowledge. Here's to our collective health and wellbeing.

This book is also dedicated to the pioneering scientists who discovered Omega-3 fatty acids. Your relentless pursuit of knowledge and understanding has opened new doors in the realm of health and nutrition. Your work has not only enlightened us about the importance of these essential fats but has also paved the way for further research and discovery. Your contributions have made a significant impact on our lives, and for that, we are profoundly grateful. This book stands as a tribute to your dedication and the lasting legacy of your scientific discovery."

This book is dedicated to all those who embark on the journey of self-discovery and health. May the knowledge within these pages inspire you to make choices that nourish not just your body, but also your soul. To the seekers, the curious, and the health-conscious—this is for you.

Foreword

In today's fast-paced world, the realm of health and nutrition can be a maze. Amidst the myriad of supplements and health trends, one crucial nutrient has been overshadowed—Omega-3 fatty acids. Collaborating with Hans-Thomas Richter on this book has enlightened me about the significance of Omega-3, not just as a buzzword, but as a cornerstone of our well-being. The economy of the last century, with its focus on extending shelf-life, has inadvertently compromised the freshness and nutritional integrity of our food. This shift, driven by food industries, has led to a noticeable decline in Omega-3 in our diets.

Historically, our ancestors consumed diets rich in Omega-3. This book delves into how economic and industrial changes have altered our food landscape, leading to an Omega-3 deficiency in modern diets. We'll explore the myriad benefits of Omega-3, from enhancing mood and health to boosting success. Instead of navigating the overwhelming world of supplements, we simplify the journey by spotlighting the profound impact of Omega-3. Embark on this enlightening journey and rediscover the essence of true health. Welcome to the revitalized world of Omega-3.

Ingemar Anderson, Publisher

Introduction

"The true sign of intelligence is not knowledge but imagination."

—Albert Einstein

In the expansive labyrinth of life's mysteries, hidden in plain sight, lies a potent entity—Omega-3 fatty acids. Like a secret code embedded in our diets, waiting to unlock boundless health benefits, this element has been the cornerstone of my lifelong odyssey, both as a scientist and an individual. But the path leading to this revelation has been far from straightforward.

This journey is not just about Omega-3 but about an understanding how the medical system, big pharma and the major food corporations have influenced nutrition and convoluted the simplest of all understandings of what we have been eating as humans and should be eating as consumers.

Indeed, the understanding of human nutrition has been deeply influenced by various factors over time, including industrial interests, cultural practices, governmental policies, and scientific research. Here are a few key points on this complex issue:

Food Industry Influence: The food and beverage industry, like any other, exists to make a profit. This can sometimes lead to practices that prioritize sales over health. For example, to make products more appealing and prolong shelf-life, companies often add sugars, unhealthy fats, and artificial ingredients to their products. These practices, along with aggressive marketing strategies, have contributed to the rise of unhealthy diets and related diseases like obesity and heart disease.

Pharmaceutical Influence: Similarly, the pharmaceutical industry has a vested interest in the treatment of disease, often through medication. While medications are deemed crucial for the Management of many health conditions, they are often over-prescribed or used in place of lifestyle changes that could address the root cause of the problem. It is therefore crucial to advocate for a holistic approach to health that includes proper nutrition and lifestyle modifications.

Government Policy and Subsidies: The policies and subsidies set by governments can greatly influence what types of food are produced and consumed. For example, in some countries, subsidies for corn and soybeans have contributed to an overproduction of these crops, which are often used to make cheap, processed foods. For that same reason many Pharmaceutical schemes are also government subsidized.

Scientific Research: Science plays a key role in shaping our understanding of nutrition. However, nutrition science can be complex to understand for the average consumer and sometimes contradictory. Unfortunately, many scientific studies are funded by food or pharmaceutical companies, which can potentially bias the results.

Public Perception and Media: The public's perception of what is healthy is greatly influenced by media and popular culture. Fashionable diets and dietary trends frequently emerge and disappear, often lacking robust scientific evidence to back their assertions. Numerous online articles might give the impression of being scientifically grounded, yet they often lack any substantiation from peer-reviewed research.

Therefore, it's important for individuals to educate themselves about nutrition and make informed food choices. Omega-3 fatty acids are a good example of a nutrient that has been shown to have numerous health benefits, but it just isn't adequately consumed in typical Western diets.

Dilemma #1: Humans rely on the consumption of grazing animals (ruminants) or cold water fish for their intake of essential Omega-3. A constant steady supply of fresh Omega-3 in our diet is essential to our health. Certainly, whole foods should provide the best nutrition.

However the reality is that we now consume massive amounts of inflammatory Omega-6 and our food is devoid of many nutrients due to the over-farming and processing, shelflife requirements, and even so-called 'natural foods' have to undergo a processing by FDA safety standards.

Dilemma #2: Natural sources of Omega-3 are simply hard to find because access to fresh (unfrozen) and wild caught fish is becoming rare and expensive. Grass-fed beef loses its Omega-3 content on the feedlot that consists mainly of grain. Farm raised poultry or pork is also usually fed a grain rich diet which results in a high inflammatory 6/3 index!

Dilemma #3: Independent testing reveals that most supplements are rancid and provide only inadequate amounts of EPA and DHA. Up to 97% of the populations, even in traditional fishing countries such as Norway and Taiwan present up to 95% Omega-3 deficient. The results show a high inflammatory index for industrial nations.

Dilemma #4: The Omega-6/3 inflammatory index has been officially adapted into medical science for decades but yet today it is not part of routine blood work. This leaves us in the dark of how to interpret other inflammatory markers in the blood !

Dilemma #5: Numerous studies on Omega-3 are conducted with supplements that are either substandard or spoiled, which leaves not only the average consumers, but also the researchers themselves, in a state of uncertainty. However, those studies that examine the consumption of fresh fish and explicitly establish the Omega-6/3 index clearly demonstrate a nearly 100% correlation between Omega-3 deficiency and inflammation, thereby establishing a connection to contemporary chronic diseases.

Dilemma #6: In addition, "the narrative against consumption of fat-rich red meats" is deeply seated. The indoctrination against cholesterol and saturated fat has little scientific bases but simply feeds into the interests of big pharma and the food industry. The production of artificial fats and meat substitutes does not take into account the inflammatory Omega-6/3 index. The problem is simply ignored.

The genesis of my personal quest dates back to 1985, at the distinguished Medical University in Hannover, Germany. As a young scientist, I had the honor of being at the forefront of groundbreaking work. Well, at that time I was simply a new student learning the basic narrative and the research was likely not related to good nutrition but the discovery of yet another cyclooxygenase-2 inhibitory drug.

However, this memorable day when I was assigned my first hands-on lab procedure on one of the earliest PC-assisted lab HPLC (High-Performance Liquid Chromatography) was a baptism of fire. Our target: inflammatory Omega-6 fatty acids. The mission was fraught with challenges of crashing computers and struggles to produce results, but nevertheless the beginning of a crusade that shaped my scientific vision and my fascination with the complexities of the human body.

Today, 35 years into my journey, my fascination with Omega-3 is as strong as ever. It's no longer an obscure scientific concept but a powerful tool that is changing lives daily in my clinical practice. I now have found freedom on this journey—the freedom of knowledge, the freedom to challenge the status quo, and most importantly, the freedom to offer a beacon of hope to those navigating the often stormy waters of health and wellbeing.

As the years unfurled, my scientific journey would continue its course, winding through the intricate terrains of cellular membranes and protein science. We were like explorers on a grand expedition, our compass pointing toward a pioneering goal: solving one of the first membrane protein crystal structures at high resolution. But the stakes were high; we were venturing into a realm that demanded not only precision but also creativity. To unravel the enigma of atomic positions, we had to weave lipid-fats directly into the protein structure—a daring and innovative approach that would be the crowning achievement of our endeavors in understanding how the cellular membranes work.

Yet, despite these accomplishments and the profound insights into biological intricacies they brought, a critical piece of the puzzle seemed to elude me. For all my knowledge and experience, the full spectrum of Omega-6 and Omega-3 fatty acids' importance for the human body remained shrouded in mystery. Like a beautifully crafted cipher, it was there, embedded in decades of research and understanding, yet I remained blissfully unaware of its profundity.

Time has a fascinating way of unveiling truths. It was not until recently, as I delved deeper into the core existential question— What is the definition of life?—that the relevance of Omega-3 began to emerge from the shadows. To my surprise, I unearthed a startling revelation: Omega-3 is not just a mere participant in the body's functions. It is a crucial catalyst, influencing every process and leaving an indelible imprint on our overall health and well-being.

In essence, Omega-3 is like the grand master in a game of chess, silently orchestrating moves, influencing outcomes, and ultimately determining the state of the game—our health. My journey led me to understand that it's not just about the presence of Omega-3 in our diets; it's about understanding how its deficiency or abundance can significantly tip the scales of our health, happiness, and success.

In the grand theater of life, the stage is set in an unlikely place—the 'lipid rafts' of the cell membrane. These tiny, dynamic territories in our cells are where vital biochemical exchanges occur, orchestrating life as we know it. The realization hit me like a bolt of lightning in the middle of a stormy night striking Huckleberry Finn sitting on a raft floating down the Mississippi river — "No Omega- 3, no life."

Indeed, the roles of Omega-3 are as myriad as the stars in the night sky. These fatty acids are the unsung heroes maintaining the fluidity and function of these lipid rafts, essentially underpinning life itself. And yet, our modern diets have cast Omega-3 into the shadows, favoring their Omega-6 counterparts much like the way the modern farming societies of the last 10,000 years favored grain over the over the free-spirited fishing and hunting mentality of Huckleberry Finn.

This imbalance, this departure from nature's intended equilibrium, has unshackled a plethora of chronic civilization diseases. We're plagued by ailments that, in ancient times, were as unfamiliar as a cell phone or a jet plane.

The question that then looms before us, like a mighty river barge in the fog, is why have we not heard of this silent crisis? It is as if society is floating down a river, oblivious to the fact that we're heading towards a waterfall. Why isn't the Omega-6/Omega-3 balance test the gold standard in blood tests, lighting our path like the lighthouse on the riverbank?

Just as Copernicus revolutionized the cosmos's understanding, the time has come for us to shift our perspective on health and nutrition. Much like many heroes of the past that changed the course of history, we must muster the courage to challenge established norms and venture towards the truth, however unsettling it may be. The stakes are high, but the reward is the promise of a healthier, more vibrant life, guided by the wisdom of Omega-3. Our adventure into the world of these essential fats is just beginning.

The science on Omega-3 research is solid and I am now convinced Omega-3 is the most important nutraceutical! A typical busy adult can only focus on a few supplements to add to his daily regimen, so choose them wisely!

The Omega-3 dilemma started when Humans "grew up" depending on either grass fed meat or cold water fatty fish for 200,000 years. Farming came much later and even then domesticated meat became the staple food. Somehow humans knew that they can only convert very little Alpha-linolenic acid into vital EPA and DHA. Modern blood tests now reveal that almost nothing gets converted at older age so humans end up over 90% deficient in many cases.

This book goes beyond merely discussing the crucial role of Omega-3 in our bodies. We will delve into the critical examination of the fats and oils deemed 'safe' for consumption in our modern-day diets. As we uncover the realities of our dietary habits, we will explore the wide range of oils available in the market, from the commonly used, such as olive and canola oils, to the lesser-known but equally important ones, such as flaxseed and chia seed oils.

An area of particular concern that we will address is the issue of rancidity in Omega-3 supplements. Omega-3 fatty acids, especially in supplement form, are prone to oxidation, leading to rancidity. Consuming rancid oils not only deprives us of the health benefits of Omega-3 but can also introduce harmful compounds into our bodies.

We aim to equip you with the necessary knowledge to navigate the complex world of dietary fats. The Omega-3 Dilemma provides you with practical guidelines for selecting oils and Omega-3 supplements, ensuring that you obtain the maximum health benefits while avoiding potential pitfalls. By understanding the complexities of these essential nutrients, we can make more informed decisions that promote optimal health and well-being.

In the early 2000s, the Omega-6/3 index emerged as a valuable tool for assessing an individual's inflammatory status. Despite its potential to offer critical insights into one's overall health, this simple blood test has yet to become a routine part of standard blood exams. Furthermore, Western medical care has not adapted the Omega-6/3 index as an essential indicator of health and inflammation. This book attempts to dive into the reasons behind this apparent neglect and aims to raise awareness about the importance of understanding and monitoring our Omega-6/3 ratio. By examining the historical and social factors that have shaped our dietary habits and medical practices, we can better comprehend the challenges in embracing this crucial marker of health.

We will explore the potential benefits of incorporating the Omega-6/3 index into routine medical care, as well as the steps that can be taken to encourage its widespread adoption. As we navigate the often-confusing world of nutrition and health, this book seeks to empower individuals with the knowledge to make informed decisions about their diet and lifestyle, ultimately promoting a healthier future for all.

Much later the uncharted path of my journey led me to the wisdom of the East and I found myself delving into the depths of Traditional Chinese Medicine (TCM). Just like the interweaving rivulets of the mighty Mississippi, my fascination with the human body's microcosmic intricacies started weaving into the rich tapestry of TCM's holistic philosophy. It was here that the concept of balance, epitomized in the principles of Yin and Yang, brought a new perspective to my understanding of fats.

In TCM, the body is seen as a balanced, interconnected system, a microcosm that mirrors the macrocosm of the universe. Foods, like the body's elements, are categorized as either Yin or Yang. However, the Yin and Yang of fats was something that ancient texts did not emphasize. Perhaps, it was because, in the early years, they had abundant access to a balanced diet. They lived closer to the earth, consumed foods that were nourished by natural resources, their meals brimming with essential nutrients.

Fast forward to our current times, we're faced with a peculiar conundrum — being 'overfed yet undernourished.' Our food system has undergone a dramatic transformation over the last 50 years. Mass production, industrial farming, and processing have robbed our foods of their vitality. Tests reveal that up to 80% of the essential nutrients are missing from our modern diets.

More alarming is the realization that we are throwing away a staggering two-thirds of every dollar we spend on food. How so, you may wonder. The answer lies in our body's ability to absorb nutrients. Devoid of essential nutrients, particularly the life-sustaining Omega-3, our body struggles to extract and utilize the sparse nutrition from the foods we eat.

We are by design visual people and our much increased time on the screen now literally requires every last DHA molecule available to the eye, because the retina always has priority. The result is that at an Omega-3 deficiency of up to 95% there is little DHA left over for other vital brain and heart functions.

As I pen this introduction, a quote "Sometimes, a change of perspective is all it takes to see the light again." comes to mind. My perspective on Omega-3 has certainly transformed my life and strength, and I invite you, dear reader, to embark on this fascinating journey with me. Together, we will explore the power of Omega-3, uncovering its influence on our lives, and unlocking a world of benefits hidden in plain sight. Here's to a journey of discovery, of understanding, and ultimately, of health transformation.

Ωm3ga

Chapter 1

Discovering Omega-3

1.1 Your Secret Superfood

In the intricate tapestry of human nutrition, one nutraceutical has shone consistently, illuminating our understanding of the pivotal role in human health: Omega-3 fatty acids. As of July 2023, in a search on the Public National Library of Medicine on the topic of "Omega-3," over 37,000 scientific publications appear [2].

Research on Omega-3, which piques the clinical interests of thousands of researchers globally, spans topics from Alzheimer's to the Zoster virus. A search on "nutrition" on amazon book titles yields over 60,000 titles and ~2,000 titles focus on "fish oil" but almost none on "Omega-3" as part of the title.

After decades of research and clinical studies all the findings are painting a clear picture: Omega-3 is probably the most important nutraceutical humans need to be healthy. Among many names in Omega-3 research Dr. Artemis P. Simopoulos stands out, a relentless sentinel in the domain of Omega-3 research. In the cryptic, mysterious world of nutritional science, her work has been nothing short of a beacon.

Dr. Simopoulos embarked on her Omega-3 exploration journey in 1965, a time when the global consciousness was barely stirring the profound implications of dietary choices on health. With the persistence of a seasoned detective and the acuity of a scholar, she plunged into the labyrinth of nutritional biochemistry. Her objective was crystal clear—to unearth the hidden truths of Omega-3 fatty acids and decode their far-reaching influence on human well-being.

Her tireless efforts have produced over 130 publications [3], each one a testament to her dedication and an invaluable addition to our collective knowledge. These publications are not just articles or research papers; they are a constellation of insights that have enriched the conversation around Omega-3 and Omega-6 fatty acids. This body of work is akin to a map charting unexplored territories, providing invaluable directions for scientists, nutritionists, and health enthusiasts around the globe and her 1999 book "The Omega Diet: The Lifesaving Nutritional Program" stands out.

Dr. Simopoulos's research has had a particular emphasis on the importance of balance. Like the harmonious yin and yang of ancient philosophy, her work underscores the need for a symbiotic balance between Omega-3 and Omega-6 fatty acids in our diet. The balance, she argues, is not an optional luxury but a critical necessity. It's akin to the perfectly synchronized gears of an intricate timepiece, each contributing to the smooth, unerring passage of time, or in this case, the optimal functioning of our bodies.

Unraveling the mysteries of this delicate equilibrium, Dr. Simopoulos has painted a fascinating picture of the biochemical dance that occurs within our bodies. She explains how the imbalance of these fatty acids—often leaning towards an overconsumption of Omega-6 and the scarcity of Omega-3—can throw our health off balance. Her research is not just a scientific revelation but a clarion call to reassess our dietary habits and shift towards an Omega-3-rich diet.

In the realm of Omega-3 fatty acids, Dr. Simopoulos is akin to a famed symbologist, deciphering complex codes and revealing profound truths hidden within. She makes sense of the convoluted and translates it into the understandable, all with a singular focus—enhancing our knowledge and encouraging healthier dietary choices. Her work is an invitation, calling us to partake in the bounty of benefits offered by Omega-3.

As we delve into the world of Omega-3, Dr. Simopoulos's work and many others will serve as our guide, our reference, and our compass. It is through her pioneering discoveries that we can fully appreciate the magnitude of Omega-3's influence on our health, happiness, and success. Many other researchers can be named here such as Mozaffarian who has dedicated his career to Omega-3, nutrition and heart disease for over 2 decades with over 530 publications [129].

Embarking on this journey, let's remember a sentiment from Dan Brown's 'The Da Vinci Code': "The only difference between you and God is that you have forgotten you are divine." So too, in the case of Omega-3—its divinity in our diet is merely forgotten. And it's high time we remembered.

As we ride this riveting river of health exploration, it's essential to look back at the origins of our modern dietary habits. We cannot fully comprehend the health implications of our current food choices without understanding the historical shifts in our diet. Researchers Watkins and Cordain provide a crucial compass in their seminal paper, "Origins and evolution of the Western diet: health implications for the 21st century." [4]

Period	Calories from fat (%)	Omega-6 intake (g/day)	Omega-3 intake (g/day)	Trans-fat intake (g/day)	Total Fat intake (g/day)
50,000 years ago	30-35	2-3	2-3	Negligible	50-60
5,000 years ago	25-30	4-5	2-3	Negligible	60-70
1800	20-25	5-7	1-2	Negligible	70-80
1900	30-35	8-10	0.5-1.5	Negligible	80-100
1950	35-40	10-15	0.5-1	1-2	90-110
2000	35-40	15-20	0.1-0.5	2-5	100-120

Table.: Table of Historic Human Fat Intace: Fat, fatty acid (Omega-6, Omega-3, trans, and total) intake (as percent of calories from fat; hypothetical extrapolation). Data were extrapolated from cross-sectional analyses of contemporary hunter-gatherer populations; [5]

The evolution of the human diet has been influenced by many factors, including availability of food, development of agriculture, industrialization, and changes in lifestyle. However, please note that the exact numbers for these eras are hard to ascertain, and the following statements are estimated values based on available research:

1. The figures of human fat consumption are general estimates and vary greatly among different populations and dietary habits.

2. Trans-fat intake has increased in recent decades due to the widespread use of partially hydrogenated oils in processed foods.

3. Omega-6 intake has risen due to increased consumption of vegetable oils and processed foods, while Omega-3 intake has decreased due to lower consumption of fish and seafood.

4. It's assumed that during the Paleolithic era (50,000 years ago), humans had a more balanced Omega-6 to Omega-3 ratio, possibly even 1:1. Today, the ratio in typical Western diets is estimated to be over 20:1.

5. The increase in total fat intake over the years has been largely due to increases in saturated and trans-fat, while unsaturated fat intake has remained relatively stable.

Much like a young hero, they courageously navigate through the foggy waters of our dietary past. They meticulously trace back the evolution of our diet from the times of our hunter-gatherer ancestors to the neolithic agricultural revolution [6] and finally the modern Western diet of processed foods. Their findings paint a stark picture of our drastic dietary deviation from nature, much like a nomads' perilous departure from his nurturing river to the corrupted societies onshore.

As we delve into the details of the Watkins and Cordain study, the correlation between the Western diet and so-called 'diseases of civilization' comes to the fore. Just as many past revolutionaries were exposed to the unjust societal norms of their time, we too are victims of a dietary shift that has fueled the rise of chronic illnesses.

In the murky waters of today's food industry, it's the high intake of Omega-6 fatty acids and the deficiency of Omega-3 fatty acids that pose a significant health risk. This imbalance is integrally connected to the societal imbalances in the poverty stricken population of all ages. It has been linked to diseases such as heart disease, diabetes, obesity, and even mental health disorders.

But there is hope. Just as Huckleberry Finn in Mark Twain's story used his resourcefulness and wit to navigate through his challenging journey of injustice on the Mississippi river, YOU too can steer our health ship towards safer shores. The insights offered by Watkins and Cordain's research point towards a solution – rebalancing our Omega-6 to Omega-3 ratio to mimic that of our ancestors.

In the grand epic of our health journey, understanding the origins and evolution of the Western diet is akin to understanding the undercurrents that shape the course of the Mississippi. As we forge ahead, let's arm ourselves with this knowledge and take active steps towards healthier food choices, just as many heroes did when they sought freedom and justice. As we take on this journey, let us remember that, like Huck, we too possess the courage, resilience, and spirit needed to triumph over the health challenges of our time to make the right decisions for our diet.

1.2 Why Omega-3 Matters

Simple Benefits

Every story has a HEART, a core that imbues it with life, character, and meaning. In the narrative of our health nothing is more important than Your Heart health and Omega-3 fatty acids play a very central role. A benevolent agent in a clandestine mission, Omega-3 silently ensures the well-being of our most vital organ, OUR HEART. Like the faithful pulse that beats within our chest, Omega-3 carries out its tasks unobtrusively, yet its role is paramount in maintaining our heart health.

Imagine Omega-3 as an unsung hero, tirelessly working behind the scenes. It aids in reducing levels of triglycerides, harmful fats in our bloodstream that can lead to atherosclerosis, and by extension, heart disease. Omega-3 also has the potential to lower blood pressure and heart rate, orchestrating a symphony of benefits for our cardiovascular system. It's as if this superfood holds the key to a lock guarding our heart health.

Beyond the heart, Omega-3 also performs an equally vital role for our brain. It's like the mastermind behind the scenes, ensuring the smooth functioning of our cognitive processes. Omega-3's importance in brain health cannot be overstated. It supports memory, attention, and other cognitive functions. In essence, it's akin to the architect of the neural pathways that shape our thoughts, actions, and behaviors.

As we age, the threat of dementia looms like a menacing specter. Here too, Omega-3 offers a ray of hope. Picture it as a guardian of our neural integrity, providing an added layer of protection against neurodegenerative disorders like Alzheimer's disease. By maintaining brain health, Omega-3 contributes significantly to preserving our cognitive abilities, allowing us to age with grace and mental agility.

Then there's the colossal challenge of "metabolic syndrome diseases"—a modern-day epidemic sweeping across the globe. Omega-3, however, stands firm in this battle. It steps in like a vigilant sentinel, helping to regulate metabolism and fight metabolic syndromes like obesity and diabetes. It's as if Omega-3 carries the torch that lights our way through the treacherous labyrinth of metabolic disorders.

But perhaps one of Omega-3's most impressive feats is its ability to combat inflammation. It's like a secret agent embedded within our immune system, countering harmful inflammation and promoting healing. By reducing inflammation, Omega-3 helps to mitigate a host of health issues, including chronic pain, autoimmune diseases, and even certain types of cancer [7,8,9,10].

The multi-faceted role of Omega-3 in our health draws parallels with the recurring theme of duality of yin and yang. Just as light and dark, science and religion, art and technology intersect in the stories of disease and nutrition, so too do the various aspects of Omega-3's benefits come together to paint a comprehensive picture of health and vitality.

Metabolic Disease and Omega-3 deficiency

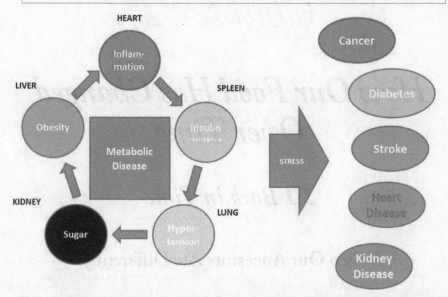

Fig. 1: Chronic civilization disease can be summed up under the umbrella of metabolic disease. These diseases are all connected through the root of Omega-3 deficiency, causing massive chronic inflammation.

So, why does Omega-3 matter? The answer, dear reader, lies in its sweeping influence on the health of every stem cell in our bodies, much like the hidden threads woven into the tapestry of a mystery novel, subtly shaping its narrative. Omega-3 is a silent guardian, a powerful ally, and a true superfood nutraceutical. And this is our quest—to understand, appreciate, and harness the power of this remarkable nutrient for our collective health and well-being.

Chapter 2

How Our Food Has Changed Over Time

2.1 Back in Time

When Our Ancestors Ate Differently

Like a well-preserved relic from a forgotten era, our ancestral diet holds intriguing secrets about our health and well-being. Time may have weathered the tangible traces of our forebears' lifestyle, but it has failed to erase their nutritional wisdom. In this age of convenience and surplus, it's worth taking a leaf out of our ancestors' book, especially when it comes to the intake of essential fatty acids.

The evidence comes from scientists that have dedicated their research for decades to this topic: Dr. Artemis Simopoulos, and her early comprehensive research paper "Essential Fatty Acids in Health and Chronic Disease" [5] and Loren Cordain "Origins and evolution of the Western diet" [4]. Both painted a vivid picture of our ancestors' dietary patterns. They took us on a journey back in time, into the dietary habits of our predecessors, whose meals were a far cry from the ones we are accustomed to today.

Imagine stepping into a time machine, winding the clock back thousands of years. Our ancestors led a life immersed in nature, where their meals were sourced from the land and sea around them. Their diet had a significantly different ratio of Omega-6 to Omega-3 fatty acids than what we find in our modern meals. It was a balanced symphony of 1-2:1, a nutritional harmony that contributed to their overall health and vitality.

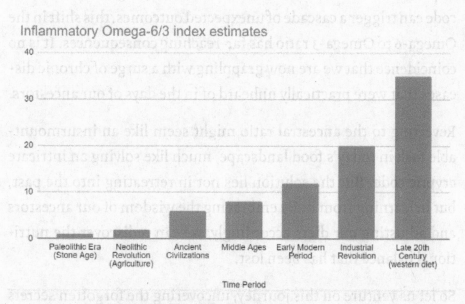

Fig. 2.: In the history of human evolution, the Inflamatory Index has increased from 1:1 to 35:1. [12]

Fast forward to the present day, and the landscape of our diet has changed drastically. Like an ancient code altered beyond recognition, the balance of Omega-6 and Omega-3 in our diets has been severely distorted. Today, in Western diets, the ratio has escalated to a staggering 20-100:1. It's as if we've strayed from a well-charted path, into an unknown terrain fraught with health challenges.

But how did we find ourselves so far adrift from our nutritional roots? The answer lies in the subtle but consistent shifts in our dietary habits over the centuries. As civilization advanced, our diets began to favor foods high in Omega-6 fatty acids. Agricultural advancements and industrialization further skewed our diet towards Omega-6 rich grains and oils.

This transition, while perhaps seemingly benign, has had profound implications on our health. Just as a minor change in an intricate code can trigger a cascade of unexpected outcomes, this shift in the Omega-6 to Omega-3 ratio has far-reaching consequences. It is no coincidence that we are now grappling with a surge of chronic diseases that were practically unheard of in the days of our ancestors.

Reverting to the ancestral ratio might seem like an insurmountable task in today's food landscape, much like solving an intricate cryptic code. But the solution lies not in retreating into the past, but in learning from it. By embracing the wisdom of our ancestors and adjusting our diets accordingly, we can rediscover the nutritional balance that has been lost.

So let us venture on this journey, uncovering the forgotten secrets of our ancestral diet, and finding our way back to a healthier Omega-6 to Omega-3 ratio. It is, after all, a quest for our health, and a step closer to understanding the intricate relationship between our food and well-being.

Consider the staggering statistics drawn from over a million inflammatory test results across the western world. The numbers paint a picture not unlike a meticulously constructed plotline, where every element subtly influences the outcome.

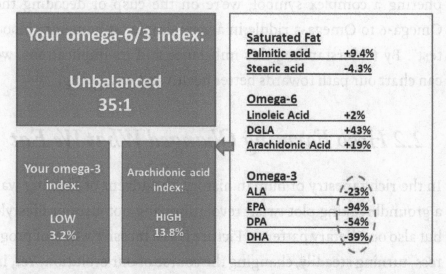

Typical Omega-6/3 Fatty Acid Test Result

Your omega-6/3 index:

Unbalanced
35:1

Your omega-3 index:

LOW
3.2%

Arachidonic acid index:

HIGH
13.8%

Saturated Fat	
Palmitic acid	+9.4%
Stearic acid	-4.3%
Omega-6	
Linoleic Acid	+2%
DGLA	+43%
Arachidonic Acid	+19%
Omega-3	
ALA	-23%
EPA	-94%
DPA	-54%
DHA	-39%

Fig. 3: A typical US test is above 30:1 and even fishing countries like Norway and Japan are testing above 10:1; desired is an index lower than 4:1.

The average inflammatory test results in the western world make for a sobering read. The ratio of Omega-6 to Omega-3, a critical factor in inflammation, stands alarmingly high at over 25:1. It's as if a cryptic imbalance, silently woven into the fabric of our diets, is unraveling, its consequences reverberating through our collective health. [13]

Even in countries where fishing, and consequently Omega-3 intake, is prevalent, the imbalance persists [14]. Although somewhat better than the USA, in Norway and Japan, where the seas generously offer their bounty on a daily basis, the Omega-6 to Omega-3 ratio still remains well above 10:1. It's as if the ancient code of our ancestors' dietary wisdom has been tampered with across the globe, resulting in a distortion that's reflecting in our health.

These startling figures, however, are not a cul-de-sac, but a crossroads, a challenge that we're poised to meet head-on. Like deciphering a complex symbol, we're on the cusp of decoding the Omega-6 to Omega-3 riddle in a very simple "at home dry blood test". By understanding this imbalance and its implications, we can chart our path towards better health and well-being.

2.2 How Farming Changed What We Eat

In the rich tapestry of human history, the advent of farming was a groundbreaking plot twist, revolutionizing not just our lifestyle but also our dietary patterns. Picture it as a massive wheel of progress, turning steadily, changing the course of our evolution. Yet, in its relentless march, farming has subtly reshaped our diets, transforming the balance of essential nutrients, especially the Omega-3 fatty acids.

It's as if we've stumbled into a vast labyrinth, one that veils the truth of our food supply's gradual depletion of Omega-3. Amid the array of tantalizing foods offered by modern agriculture, we have lost sight of the nutritional powerhouse that is Omega-3. Ultra-processed foods, replacing traditional meals, serve as the perfect decoy, distracting us from the nutrient imbalance they carry within.

Our dietary detour does not stop at processed foods. Even our choices of meats have been swayed from the path our ancestors walked. Once, red meat sourced from grass-fed animals was a prime provider of Omega-3, akin to a hidden clue leading us towards optimal health. Today, however, it's a different story. Our preference for grain-fed meat has silently yet significantly eroded the Omega-3 content in our diet.

The same narrative unfolds in our seafood choices. Cold water fish, nature's very own Omega-3 treasure chests, have gradually vanished from our plates. As we move further away from these rich sources, it's as though we're walking away from a vital clue, one that holds the key to unlock our health potential.

Adding to this conundrum are the foods advertised as Omega-3 rich—nuts, oils, and the like. They appear to be guiding us back to our Omega-3 roots, but here lies the twist. These foods, while indeed housing Omega-3, also carry a high Omega-6 content. It's as if they're a cryptic trap, housing a secret within a secret, an Omega-3 promise wrapped in an Omega-6 enigma.

This shift in our diets, driven by modern farming practices, mirrors the multi-layered conspiracies that drive the narratives in a crime novel. Beneath the surface of food abundance lies the hidden plot of Omega-3 depletion, quietly influencing our health outcomes.

Indeed, the journey to optimal Omega-3 intake might appear as enigmatic and convoluted as the plotline of Dostoevsky's crime and punishment. Picture the average person, striving to navigate the maze-like landscape of online nutrition information with its 60,000 books and 100,000s publications. It's akin to finding oneself in an expansive library, lined with countless volumes of nutrition advice, each contradicting the other.

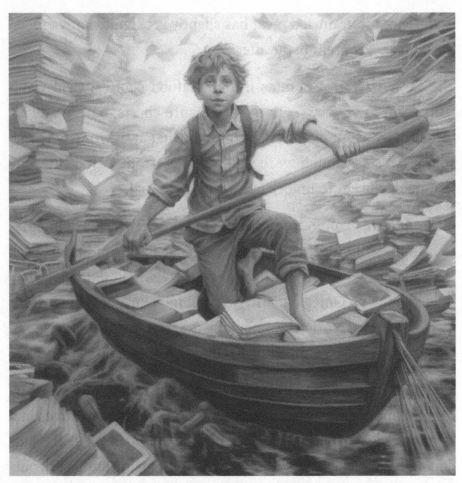

Fig. 4: Navigating through 60,000+ books on nutrition

The path is fraught with misleading claims, unverified advice, and complex dietary protocols, mirroring the array of deceptive clues in a fiction novel. Take for example the entire discussion around Cholesterol, triglycerides and fatty red meats. Just as an experienced scientist tries to navigate through baffling symbols and hidden truths, the average person must decipher the tangled web of online nutrition guidance. Yet, much like Simopoulos unswerving efforts to resolve and unlock the truth, we too must press on undeterred and question the narrative.

At times, the truth about Omega-3 can seem as elusive as the Holy Grail. So many sources boast high Omega-3 content, only for their claims to be overshadowed by equally high or higher Omega-6 content. However this puzzle, a riddle wrapped in an enigma is easier to understand than one might believe.

Every mystery, no matter how confounding, carries within it the potential for revelation. The quest for optimal Omega-3 intake is no different. You too can piece together the scattered fragments of truth to form a coherent, beneficial picture of Omega-3 nutrition. Though the path is fraught with misinformation and misdirection, with tenacity and discernment, we can separate the wheat from the chaff. Like a keen-eyed symbologist deciphering an intricate code, we can learn to identify and understand valid, scientifically supported information amid the cacophony of online nutritional advice.

In this labyrinth of nutrition information, our compass is scientific research, guiding us towards accurate and beneficial knowledge. And just like any adventure, our quest for the truth about Omega-3 intake, while challenging, promises to be a rewarding and enlightening journey much like Huckleberry Finn's adventures on his raft.

The path back to optimal Omega-3 intake might seem shrouded in mystery. Yet, just as every code can be deciphered, every challenge can be overcome. By peeling back the layers of our dietary choices and understanding the influence of farming practices, we can begin to rewrite our nutritional narrative.

Thus begins our journey, retracing the path back to Omega-3 richness, armed with knowledge, intent, and a resolve to rediscover the nutritional balance of our ancestors. It's a quest, much like the thrilling adventures of Huckleberry Finn, that promises revelations, challenges, and ultimately, a triumphant return to health and well-being.

Indeed, the quest for optimal Omega-3 intake can be compared to the thrilling adventures of Huckleberry Finn. Each of us embarks on this journey with an exploratory spirit, akin to the young, adventurous Huck, navigating the vast and sometimes daunting river of nutritional information.

Just as Huck faced numerous trials and tribulations, we too encounter myriad challenges. We confront misleading information, just as Huck confronted the cunning schemes of the conmen, the "Duke and the King" narrative of western nutrition. We battle the confusion of contradicting advice, similar to Huck's struggle with the moral and societal conflicts of his era. But just as Huck's adventures tested his courage and resilience, our journey tests our resolve to find the truth and achieve optimal health.

Throughout his journey, Huck experienced revelations that shaped his understanding of the world and his place in it. Similarly, as we wade through the vast river of nutritional advice, we uncover essential truths about Omega-3, saturated fat and cholesterol and its vital roles in our health. Each piece of valid information we glean is a revelation, opening our eyes to the importance of fat as the crucial nutrient.

And finally, just like Huck's story culminates in a triumphant realization of freedom and understanding, our quest too promises a triumph. It's a triumph over misinformation and confusion, a victorious return to health and well-being. As we discern the truth about Omega-3 and adjust our dietary choices accordingly, we reclaim control over our health.

So, let us embrace this quest with the spirit of Huckleberry Finn, armed with curiosity, resilience, and an unwavering desire for truth. For it's a journey that promises to be as enlightening as it is beneficial, leading us towards health and well-being. Much like Huck's adventurous voyage, it's a journey worth undertaking.

2.3 The Modern Plate: Are We Missing Out on Omega-3?

Unraveling the mysteries of our modern diet is like standing on the threshold of a bad B-movie plot, with unexpected turns, hidden truths, and revelations that both intrigue and enlighten. Could it be that our culinary landscape, as diverse and tempting as it may appear, is leading us astray in our pursuit of Omega-3?

Consider, for example, our unwitting consumption of vegetable oils. Picture the average American, unknowingly consuming up to 15 spoons of vegetable oils daily, akin to consuming more than 300g of sunflower seeds. It's a staggering statistic that flips the narrative, much like a cheap soap opera upending our understanding with a plot twist.

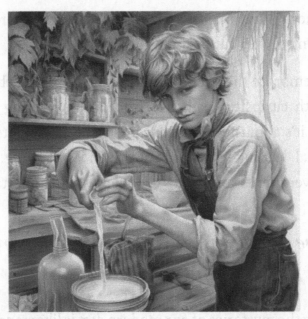

Fig. 5.: Huckleberry Finn would have never cooked with vegetable oil

This phenomenon is a product of our times, a testament to the power of modern industrial processing. Yet, much like a clandestine organization in a tale, operating in the shadows, this modern marvel may be leading us away from our desired destination of balanced nutrition.

This abundance of vegetable oils in our diets could, theoretically, be a boon. Rapeseed oil, for instance, holds the potential for hepatoprotection due to the presence of beneficial micronutrients like polyphenols, tocopherols, and phytosterols. Just as ancient symbols, these micronutrients could lead to a treasure and better health.

However, much like a key plot point obscured until the final chapters, these potential benefits are often erased by the traditional refining process. The lack of micronutrients leave us with a product that is far removed from its natural state. It's as if we're deciphering a coded message, only to find that the most crucial part of the code has been erased.

This leaves us with a quandary as intricate as a thriller best written by giant Food companies that own the production chain. If the very oils we consume in abundance are stripped of their beneficial nutrients and leave us laden with Omega-6, how can we hope to balance our Omega-3 intake?

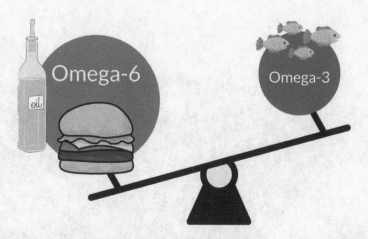

Fig. 6: The imbalance of Omega-6/3 in our current diet.

Yet, as any fan of a good Hitchcock movie would attest, no puzzle is too complex, no code too scary to solve. Our dietary puzzle is no different. By understanding the inner workings of our food supply, by unraveling the refining process and its implications, we are charting a course towards a solution.

So let's take a leaf from Copernicus book "De revolutionibus orbium coelestium" and question the status quo, challenge the foundations of our dietary universe much as Copernicus and Kepler helped question the geocentric worldview. By exploring beyond the established narrative, by embracing the unexpected, we can illuminate the nutritional cosmos surrounding us, and usher in a new era of dietary understanding and balance.

Delving into the conundrum of our modern diet is akin to embarking on an adventure as thrilling as Huckleberry Finn's journey down the Mississippi. The question looms like an uncharted island on our horizon: is our modern plate, despite its array of diverse and tempting dishes, shortchanging us on Omega-3?

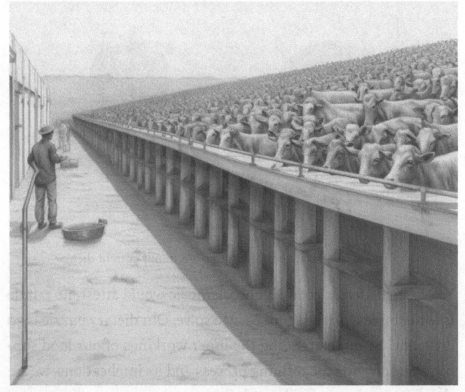

Fig. 7: Today, grass-fed cows on a feed lot lose most of Omega-3 content. [15]

Consider grass-fed beef, for example. There was a time when it was a trusted source of Omega-3, a vital nutrient tucked away within our meals, much like a hidden treasure on one of Huck's river islands. Yet, in a perplexing turn of events, today's grass-fed beef seems to have drifted away from this treasure and cows are placed for weeks on a grain-feed-lot before slaughter. This procedure causes them to lose up to ¾ of their lifetime accumulated storage of Omega-3. [15]

In a move reminiscent of Huck's unexpected detours, even grass-fed cattle often find themselves on feedlots before slaughter. Their diet shifts dramatically, transforming the nutritional landscape of the meat they provide. The once Omega-3-rich beef now contributes to the Omega-6 glut in our diets.

Meanwhile, our seafood supply, once teeming with fish fresh from the wild, has witnessed a similar shift. Wild fish, free as Huck himself, have been replaced by fish raised in restrictive farms. The resultant farmed fish still offer Omega-3, but they fall short of the nutritional bounty that their wild counterparts provide.

The combined effect of these changes presents us with a conundrum worthy of a Mark Twain novel. With both our meat and fish—our once reliable sources of Omega-3—seeing a dip in their Omega-3 content, how do we meet our dietary needs for this essential nutrient?

Yet, just as Huck found solutions to his challenges on the river, we too can find a way out of our dietary predicament. By understanding the intricacies of our food supply and acknowledging the shifts in Omega-3 content, we are already navigating our way towards an answer.

Our modern plate might be currently light on Omega-3, but the story doesn't have to end there. Just as Huck questioned societal norms, we can question and demand changes in farming practices. By seeking genuinely Omega-3-rich sources, we can influence what lands on our plates.

So, let's embrace this challenge with the spirit of Huckleberry Finn, navigating our way back to a more balanced Omega-3 intake. It's an exciting voyage, one that promises to be as thrilling as Huck's journey down the mighty Mississippi and as rewarding as the discovery of the lost treasure of health and well-being.

Plant Foods	ALA (mg)	Omega-6 (mg)	Omega-6/3 Ratio
Flaxseeds	22813	5777	0.25
Chia seeds	17552	5785	0.33
Walnuts	9079	38092	4.20
Hemp seeds	2289	23866	10.42
Canola oil	9179	19962	2.17
Soybean oil (unhydrogenated)	6801	50052	7.36
Purslane	4000	1000	0.25
Perilla oil	14928	3976	0.27
Camelina oil	10200	9600	0.94
Walnut oil	1400	57800	41.29
Mustard oil	1173	18400	15.69
Algal oil (varies)	300-2000	100-500	0.17-1.67

Table: Common plant foods rich in ALA (Alpha-linolenic acid) and their corresponding inflammatory index [16] (note: ALA has to be enzymatically converted to EPA and DHA in the body).

Just as Huck sought freedom from his restrictive and abusive life, so too we find ourselves yearning for a release from the constraints imposed upon us by a labyrinth of powerful entities. The FDA, big pharma, giant corporations, fast food chains—these are the contemporary captains of our ship, steering us down a river fraught with health hazards.

Huck's story was set against the backdrop of a society grappling with moral dilemmas and deep-seated prejudices. We, too, are participants in a narrative dominated by vast and seemingly insurmountable structures, where our dietary freedoms are being impinged upon, our access to nutritious foods limited, and our health compromised.

As readers, we empathized with Huck's plight. As consumers, we experience a similar discomfort, a shared desire to escape the restrictive clutches of these organizations that prioritize profit over public health. Just as Huck yearned for freedom, we long for the autonomy to make healthier dietary choices.

In our story, Omega-3 plays a pivotal role. It's our raft, our tool for navigating the turbulent waters of modern nutrition. It represents our hope for reclaiming control over our health, offering us the chance to resist the current of unhealthy dietary habits.

But, like Huck, we must exhibit courage. We must be willing to question the status quo, to confront the powerful entities that dictate our dietary landscape. We must take ownership of our nutrition, steer the raft away from processed foods and return to the source of meats that are embracing the therapeutic potential of Omega-3 and advocating for its place in our diets.

Ultimately, our journey mirrors Huck's pursuit of freedom. The freedom from disease. It's a journey that calls for resilience, for critical thinking, and above all, for a dogged determination to prioritize our health in a landscape that often seems stacked against us. But, like Huck, we have the capacity to navigate these complex waters, to advocate for change, and ultimately, to reclaim our dietary freedom.

Animal Protein	Omega-3 (grams per 100g)	Omega-6 (grams per 100g)	Omega-6/Omega-3 ratio
Grain-fed Beef	0.035	0.39	11.14
Pork	0.10	0.60	6.00
Poultry	0.11	0.25	2.27
Wild Boar	0.09	0.13	1.44
Deer	0.24	0.04	0.17
Elk	0.13	0.11	0.85
Rabbit	0.30	0.04	0.13
Grass-fed Beef	0.07	0.18	2.57

Table: Table of Omega-3 supplement facts of animal protein and their corresponding inflammatory indices (more complete Omega-3 supplements facts are shown in the appendix)

Please note that the Omega-6/3 ratios in different cuts of meat can vary. For example, the leaner cuts often have a higher ratio. And as mentioned before, the diet of the animal plays a significant role in determining the ratio. For example, grass-fed-grass-finished beef has a more favorable Omega-6/3 ratio than grain-fed beef due to the different types of grass and forage they consume. [17, 18]

In summary, the tables above show how only few foods contain valuble amounts Omega-3 and we will discuss later how cold water fish is likely the best source for EPA and DHA. Plant sources contain only ALA and very little EPA and DHA and ALA has to be enzymatically converted within the body, a process that is very inefficient. In addition as discussed later, Omega-3 is subject to rancidity and have to be consumed fresh.

Chapter 3

Omega-3 and Your Health The Fantastic Connection

3.1 A Secret Ingredient to reduce your inflammation

Offering a comprehensive account of all the metabolic functions in the body involving Omega-3 would exceed the scope of this book. Nevertheless, here's a brief overview:

- **Membrane Function and Fluidity:** The Omega-3 molecule chain, due to its flexible and curved nature, contributes to the fluidity and volume of cell membranes. This is crucial when a concave membrane structure is required for cell division. DHA, essentially, is integrated into one layer of the membrane (the bottom hemi layer), with the other layer containing more saturated fatty acid to produce a curvature. For this very reason "saturated fats" are also very important, specifically stearic acid and are shown to be essential for proper cell function. (See Fig.23 in chapter four and the Appendix).

- **Anti-inflammatory Eicosanoids:** This is a complex area but it essentially boils down to the contrast between inflammatory Omega-6 fatty acids and anti-inflammatory Omega-3. Hence the importance of maintaining the ratio of Omega-6 to Omega-3 lower than 4:1! [19]

- **Redox Potential:** An often overlooked factor is that Omega-3 readily oxidizes, hence, serving as a significant acceptor of electrons within the cell membrane. [20, 21]

- **Trans-Membrane Protein Function:** This includes the functioning of cytochrome C in the mitochondria. Approximately 50% of cardiolipin in the heart muscle lipids is accountable for meeting the high energy demands. Nerve and brain cells rely on the function of potassium channels; without DHA these channels can't open properly. Furthermore, Omega-3 aids in creating lipid rafts—functional units that allow protein complexes to communicate and maneuver. [22,23]

- **Epoxy Products:** Epoxy products from oxidized polyunsaturated fatty acids (PUFAs) possess a localized vasodilatory effect, making them vital for the health of the brain, heart, and kidneys. However, these epoxy molecules are rapidly eliminated by specific hydrolases, causing them to be short-lived. [24, 97]

- **Cellular Repair and Stem Cells:** No cell can divide and tissues cannot renew from stem cells without adequate Omega-3. Membrane curvatures and repair processes rely on asymmetric lipid bilayer structures.[25]

The Anti-inflammatory Action

What if I told you there is one blood test above all others to measure inflammation, superior to all others, capable of assessing inflammation at its very roots — a test whose results influence all other inflammation markers downstream. This is the Omega-6/3 Index.

There is no doubt anymore in the scientific community that systemic inflammation is the central basis for many chronic civilization diseases including metabolic syndrome, cardiovascular disease, dementia and cancer. There are many mechanisms of how Omega-3 works in every aspect of the body's function. However, reducing chronic inflammation is probably the most important of all! [26]

For almost every nutrient deficiency the body has fail-safe mechanisms to sustain life. Tests reveal that 97% of the population now tests 70-95% Omega-3 deficient. So what does the body do, when it can't use Omega-3 in the cell because it is not available? He replaces Omega-3 with Omega-6 and cholesterol! Unfortunately, Omega-6 (namely arachidonic acid) turns out to be highly inflammatory. When the cell sends out a message or breaks down at the end of its useful life, nature has installed a signaling mechanism where the OMEGA fatty acids are at the initial step of being involved in the so-called eicosanoid cascade. Now, since the balance of inflammation and anti-inflammation is chronically destroyed because average ratios of over 25:1 or even up to 100:1 inflammatory Omega-6 over 3, these inflammatory eicosanoids are bombarding the body. [27]

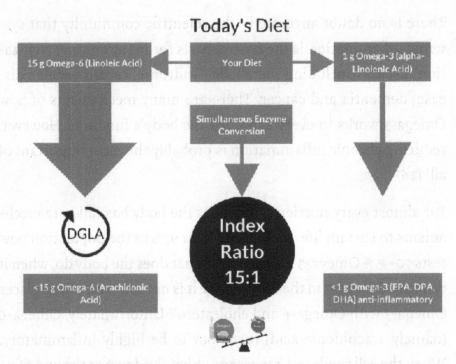

Fig. 8: Today's diet produces a high Omega-6/3 ratio (inflammatory index).

In the example avove, the ratio is 15:1. Often, the inflammatory Omega-6 called DGLA (Dihomo-Gamma-Linolenic Acid) builds up high in our bodies because the body tries to reduce excess inflammation.

Anti-inflammatory drugs like NSAIDs and aspirin work directly on this inflammatory cascade. Simply put, they inhibit the cyclooxygenase-enzymes that produce the ultimate inflammatory signaling molecules (known as PGE-series-2). From this perspective, it becomes clear that the crux of the issue lies within the imbalance of Omega-6 to Omega-3. Some level of inflammation is indeed beneficial, aiding the body in repair and renewal processes, but the presence of chronically high levels of arachidonic acids (AA) is problematic. Interestingly, the body has even established a negative feedback mechanism where the AA precursor, DGLA [31], accumulates because the body has already reached its limit.

The Secret of reducing inflammation lies within the lipid cell membrane

Immersing ourselves in the world of Omega-3 and its health benefits is akin to entering one of a thrilling tales, a world where secrets abound, revelations astound, and knowledge becomes power. So, let us unveil the mystery: Why are fish oils considered the better source for Omega-3? And what is it exactly that Omega-3 does?

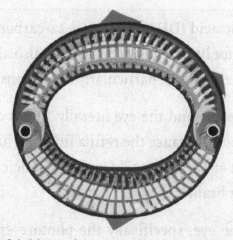

Fig. 9: Cold-water fish like sardine or mackerel are high in specific Omega-3, which increases cell-fluidity as illustrated above.

To understand this secret, we must venture beneath the surface of the cell. The realm of Omega-3 is rich and varied, but not all sources of this essential nutrient are created equal. No doubt fish oil is particularly rich in EPA [28]. Both EPA and DHA are the main players in this game, the Tiger Woods and Maradonnas of fats.

Eicosapentaenoic acid (EPA): This 20-carbon Omega-3 fatty acid is one of the most prevalent types found in fish oil. EPA is particularly known for its anti-inflammatory properties and effects on heart health.

Recent studies have shown what we have known at least since the 1960s [111] how fatty livers are affected by inflammatory Omega-6. Lands 2017: "Four weeks of fish oil supplementation caused individuals to have marked decreases in both Thromboxane and aggregation. Omega-6 ... causes healthy physiology to shift toward pathophysiology. The proportion of n-6 in tissue HUFA directly relates to the severity of conditions caused by excessive Omega-6 actions." [112]

Docosahexaenoic acid (DHA): DHA is a 22-carbon Omega-3 fatty acid that is vital for brain and eye health. It's also an essential component of cell membranes, particularly in neurons and retina.

We are visual people and the eye literally "sucks out" every available DHA molecule, because the retina function has priority. Now "imagine" if you are testing 90% Omega-3 deficient how much is left over for your brain?

The retina of the eye, specifically the photoreceptor cells in the retina, is exceptionally rich in DHA (docosahexaenoic acid), an Omega-3 fatty acid. DHA comprises over 50% of the total fatty acid content in the retina [29].

The high concentration of DHA in the retina is vital for maintaining the fluidity of photoreceptor membranes, which in turn supports the function of proteins within these membranes. These proteins are essential for photoreceptor cells to absorb light and convert it into electrical signals that the brain interprets as visual information. Thus, a deficiency in DHA can negatively impact vision and may contribute to conditions such as retinal degeneration.

Moreover, DHA also serves as a precursor to neuroprotectin D1, a molecule that has anti-inflammatory effects and protects retinal cells from oxidative stress, further underscoring the importance of DHA in eye health. [30]

Indeed, the body prioritizes the allocation of nutrients based on their relative importance to various organs and tissues. The retina is incredibly rich in DHA, one of the most important Omega-3 fatty acids. It plays a critical role in maintaining vision and eye health, so the body ensures that the retina gets a sufficient amount of DHA.

The brain is another organ that is highly dependent on Omega-3 fatty acids, particularly DHA, for its function. DHA is essential for brain health, supporting cognitive function, memory, mood, and overall mental health. A deficiency in DHA can potentially affect these aspects of brain function.

If a person's diet is severely deficient in Omega-3 fatty acids, as reflected in a very low Omega-3 index, it could potentially lead to deficiencies in both the retina and the brain. Therefore, ensuring an adequate dietary intake of Omega-3 fatty acids, either from food sources like fatty fish or through supplementation, is crucial for maintaining eye and brain health.

Fish oils emerge as the victors in this intricate plot, but what sets them apart?

Fish oils, particularly those derived from fatty fish, carry high levels of EPA and DHA, two types of Omega-3 that have been extensively studied for their health benefits. It's as if we've unearthed a treasure trove of ancient symbols, each signifying a path to better health: heart health, brain health, eye health, and more.

Yet, the plot thickens further. Fish oils being a natural product, the protagonist of our story, holds yet another secret – they harbor rare forms of Omega-3 that have not been fully studied yet. This is the fascinating realm of unknown Omega-3, the subterranean crypt where untold secrets await to be unearthed. Who knows what astounding revelations they might bring to our understanding of health and well-being?

As the whisper of an unbroken code, Indeed these undiscovered Omega-3 in fish oils present a unique opportunity. Just as the 'Catcher in the Rye' would not let an unspoken truth or an unsolved mystery rest, so too should we embrace the pursuit of knowledge. Much like the insightful yet disillusioned Holden Caulfield, we must question the accepted, look beyond the surface, and seek out the essential truths that lie hidden beneath layers of convention. This quest will lead us, not through the rye fields of life's carbohydrate illusions, but through the fertile terrain of fat-ful nutrition, revealing the truly transformative power of Omega-3.

Also remember, that fish oils are a natural product. In the light of artificially produced algae sources and Omega-3 drugs now emerging it is important to point out that we do not have a complete picture of all ingredients. Therefore in addition to the common forms of Omega-3 fatty acids (EPA, DHA, DPA, ALA), there are also several lesser-known and less abundant types. Some of these include:

Eicosatrienoic acid (ETA): An Omega-3 fatty acid that is sometimes found in fish oil. It has been less well-studied compared to EPA and DHA. [32]

Stearidonic acid (SDA): This is an 18-carbon Omega-3 fatty acid that is typically found in plant oils, but can also be found in some types of fish oil.

Heneicosapentaenoic acid (HPA): A 21-carbon Omega-3 fatty acid. It's less common than EPA, DHA, and DPA and is found in small amounts in some types of fish.

Tetracosapentaenoic acid: This is a 24-carbon Omega-3 fatty acid, also less common and found in small amounts in certain types of fish and marine oils.

Tetracosahexaenoic acid (Nisinic acid): A very long chain (24 carbons) Omega-3 fatty acid that has been found in some fish species.

However, the health benefits of these rare Omega-3 fatty acids are not as well studied as those of EPA, DHA, and ALA. Therefore, while they are present in fish oil, they're often not highlighted as a primary source of Omega-3.

What is the definition of life and what is DNA worth without its cell membrane?

As the very fabric of life, DNA, was unveiled to us through the persistent and audacious spirit of Watson and Crick. Yet, behind their groundbreaking discovery, there was an unsung hero, Rosalind

Franklin, whose Photo 51 played an instrumental role in understanding the structure of DNA [33]. They were not just exploring a molecule, but the very essence of what makes us who we are.

As the spirit of these scientific pioneers should be the north star guiding our quest to unravel the intricacies of nutrition. Like Franklin, we must be willing to dive deep and illuminate the unseen, to capture our own "photo 51" image of Omega-3. We need to expose the unseen role these essential fatty acids play in our bodies, bringing to light their profound impact on our health.

This exploration goes beyond the clinical and scientific realms. It is about illuminating societal misconceptions, the myths, and the misinformation about nutrition. This task is daunting, indeed, but just as Franklin's photographic skills were pivotal in the DNA discovery, so is our ability to present a clear and concise picture of Omega-3's role in health.

And similarly, the exploration of Omega-3 fatty acids is not just about a nutrient but the very essence of our health. 50% of the cell membrane is protein but 50% is lipids that rely on Omega-3. They actually keep each other happy and control what goes in and out of the cell. EG nerve cells channel sodium and potassium to generate an electric signal, this potassium channel relies on Omega-3 to open and close.

Omega-3 fatty acids play a vital role in our health, beyond their basic nutritional value. They are a type of polyunsaturated fat that our bodies can't produce on their own, so they must come from our diet. Let's take a closer look at how Omega-3 fatty acids contribute to our health:

Cell Membrane Health: Omega-3 fatty acids are an essential component of the phospholipids that make up the cell membranes in our bodies. They give cell membranes flexibility and integrity, which helps control the passage of substances in and out of the cells.

Neurological Function: Omega-3 fatty acids are particularly concentrated in the brain and nervous system, where they are critical for cognitive and behavioral function. Studies have shown that deficiencies in Omega-3 can lead to mood disorders, cognitive decline, and neurological abnormalities.

Heart Health: Omega-3 fatty acids have been shown to reduce inflammation, lower blood pressure, and decrease triglyceride levels, all of which contribute to heart health. They also help prevent clotting and arrhythmias, which can lead to heart attack and stroke.

Potassium Channels: Omega-3 fatty acids can directly activate large-conductance calcium-dependent potassium channels (BK channels), as pointed out by Dr. Toshinori Hoshi's research. This activity can lead to the dilation of blood vessels and the reduction of blood pressure.

Inflammation and Immunity: Omega-3 fatty acids can help reduce inflammation in the body and contribute to a well-functioning immune system. They do this by producing substances called resolvins and protectins, which have anti-inflammatory properties. [34]

These various roles make Omega-3 fatty acids an essential part of a healthy diet. Foods rich in Omega-3 include fatty fish (such as salmon, mackerel, and sardines), flaxseeds, chia seeds, walnuts, and certain types of algae. Even if these foods are not regularly consumed, test show that without supplementation a healthy inflammatory index below 4:1 cannot be achieved.

Nerve Signal Conduction needs Omega-3

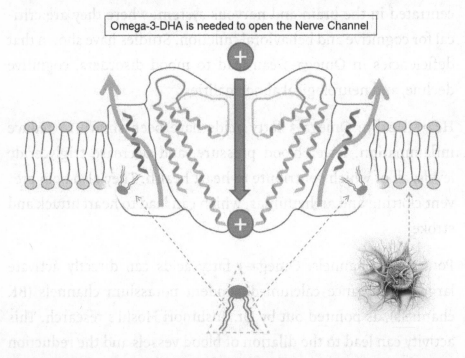

Omega-3-DHA is needed to open the Nerve Channel

Fig. 10: Schematic of an ion channel; in order to open and shuttle ions across the membrane DHA is needed for the conformation change of the outer helix. Omega-3 fatty acids lower blood pressure by directly activating large-conductance Ca2+-dependent K+ channels. Figure adapted from [35]

Indeed, lipids and membrane proteins are intimately connected in cellular biology. They are both essential components of cell membranes and interact closely with each other to ensure the proper function of the cell.

38

Membrane proteins are either embedded within the lipid bilayer or associated with its surface. Integral membrane proteins, for example, penetrate the hydrophobic core of the lipid bilayer, while peripheral membrane proteins are loosely attached to the lipid bilayer and can be easily separated from it.

The lipid environment can significantly influence the structure and function of membrane proteins. For example, specific lipids can stabilize protein structure, modulate protein function, and even facilitate protein-protein interactions. In turn, proteins can also influence the behavior of lipids in the membrane. They can cause local distortions in the lipid bilayer and affect lipid organization and dynamics.

When it comes to solving the crystal structure of membrane proteins, the role of lipids can't be overlooked. Scientists often need to include lipids in their models to obtain a more accurate picture of the protein structure. This is because the lipids can directly interact with the protein and influence its conformation.

So, to sum up, lipids and membrane proteins are highly interdependent, and their interplay is critical for the proper function of cells. Any disruptions to this relationship can have significant impacts on cellular function and could potentially lead to disease.

Lipid rafts are specialized microdomains of the plasma membrane that are enriched in cholesterol, sphingolipids, and certain proteins. They serve as organizing centers for the assembly of signaling molecules, influence membrane fluidity and membrane protein trafficking, and regulate neurotransmission and receptor trafficking.

Omega-3 fatty acids, including EPA and DHA, can be incorporated into lipid rafts and influence their composition and function. These fatty acids are known to displace cholesterol from the lipid rafts [36], leading to alterations in the raft's size, shape, and function. This displacement can influence the signaling pathways that are initiated from these rafts.

Nuclear receptors are a class of proteins found within cells that are responsible for sensing steroid and thyroid hormones and certain other molecules. These receptors, once activated, can bind to specific DNA sequences and influence the expression of nearby genes. They essentially control the "switches" that turn genes on and off.

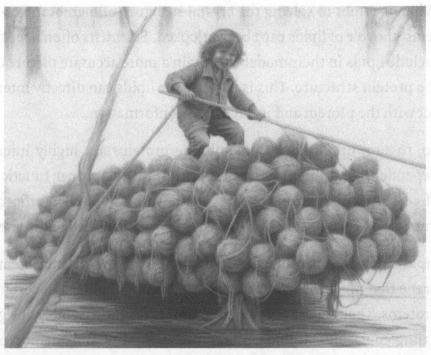

Fig. 11: Huckleberry's lipid raft.

Incorporating Omega-3 fatty acids into the lipid rafts can influence the activity of these nuclear receptors. For example, Omega-3 fatty acids are known to activate the peroxisome proliferator-activated receptors (PPARs), which are a type of nuclear receptor. Once activated, PPARs can influence the expression of genes involved in lipid metabolism, inflammation, and other processes.

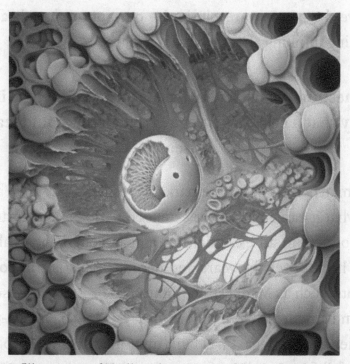

Fig. 12: Illustration of a cell nucleus protected by the lipid membrane.

So, Omega-3 fatty acids, through their incorporation into lipid rafts and interaction with nuclear receptors, can have profound effects on gene expression and cell function. It's another reason why these fatty acids are so important for our health. [37]

As we embark on this quest, let's remember the daring spirit of Watson and Crick, the persistent curiosity of Franklin, and their joint desire to illuminate life's deepest mysteries. We must step beyond the established boundaries of nutritional knowledge, daring to question, daring to explore, and daring to expose the truth.

The complex narrative of Omega-3 is waiting to be told, as is the tale of the cellular membrane and its potential impacts on health to be shared. Just as Watson, Crick, and Franklin transformed our understanding of life with the revelation of the DNA structure, we too have the power to revolutionize our approach to health and well-being thinking about what life really is.

The question persists: why has nature designed us in such a way that a critical Omega-3 deficiency could lead to disease?

The human body is indeed remarkably resilient, but there are limits to what it can endure over extended periods. A constant deficiency of 90% in an essential nutrient is bound to wreak havoc on our health over the years and decades. This is true for many nutrients, such as Magnesium, Vitamin D or B12, yet these nutrients can be replenished in hours or days. Not so Omega-3! Once a deficiency of Omega-3 has built up it may take years to replenish the full functionality of our organs. Worse, permanent damage to nerves, cardiovascular system and many organ functions is at stake here. While we may never fully understand the reasons why nature has chosen such a fragile molecule at the center of such important metabolic functions, the evolutionary connections between single-celled and multicellular organisms surely play a part. At any given moment, our bodies contain more single-cell organisms than human cells. Perhaps the creator has even installed this mechanism as a 'kill switch' to address the problem of overpopulation. Perhaps this mechanism was even installed to ensure the survival of a few fittest humans in the end stages of a world ruled by Artificial Intelligence.

Regardless of the purpose behind this obvious 'weakness', the reason humans can't directly extract EPA and DHA from algae lies in our position at the end of the food chain. As I have already discussed, in our past existence as 'hunters and gatherers,' obtaining the right amount of Omega-3 was never an issue. It's our modern lifestyle which has dramatically altered our food supply, creating the deficiency we see today.

Embracing this audacious spirit, we can further our understanding of nutrition, bringing health benefits to ourselves and future generations. We are on the brink of a nutritional revolution, poised to reveal a secret as life-changing as the double helix. Let us seize this moment and step into the light.

Indeed, the cell membrane plays a crucial role in maintaining the life of a cell. It acts as a barrier that separates the inner cell environment from the outer environment, and it is semi-permeable, allowing certain substances to pass through while keeping others out. This selective permeability is vital for the cell to get nutrients, eliminate waste, and communicate with other cells.

The cell membrane is primarily composed of a phospholipid bilayer, with the fatty acid tails of the phospholipids facing inward to form a hydrophobic region and the phosphate heads facing outward. This structure allows the membrane to be flexible and fluid. Embedded in this lipid bilayer are various proteins and other molecules that carry out specific functions such as transport, signal transduction, and cell adhesion.

Omega-3 fatty acids, such as EPA and DHA, are components of the phospholipids in the cell membrane. They contribute to the fluidity, flexibility, and function of the membrane. DHA, in particular, is highly concentrated in the membranes of cells in the brain and retina, where it plays a crucial role in neural and visual function.

In addition to contributing to membrane structure, Omega-3 fatty acids also have important roles in cell signaling and inflammation regulation. They can be converted into molecules called eicosanoids and resolvins, which have anti-inflammatory effects.

In a very real sense, Omega-3 fatty acids contribute to the 'life' of a cell by maintaining the integrity and function of the cell membrane, supporting cell signaling processes, and regulating inflammation. Without an Impeccable cell membrane, a cell would not be able to survive or carry out its functions, including DNA replication and gene expression.

Once again, all the efforts are futile without a functional cell membrane. As we navigate this fantastic connection between Omega-3 and the lipid membrane, we draw inspiration from cold water Fish, with their potent blend of known and unknown Omega-3 that keep their membranes and bodies flexible in harsh environments. As cold water fish are rich in EPA and DHA, they indeed are a secret ingredient for a healthier body, a key to a cryptex that can unlock greater well-being by making life possible.

So, let us get inspired by narratives of the Robin Hoods of true scientific heroes, from their relentless pursuit of truth, and their awe-inspiring revelations and embrace the adventure, and take a deep dive into the world of Omega-3. For it promises to be a journey as thrilling as deciphering an ancient code, and as rewarding as discovering a secret that can change our lives for the better.

3.2 Omega-3: Your Shield Against Common Illnesses

Venturing into the realm of Omega-3's protective powers against common illnesses is akin to navigating through a labyrinth of the FDAs narrative, teeming with suspense, rich in intricacy, and brimming with profound revelations. At the heart of this maze lies a critical understanding: the simultaneous intake of high EPA and DHA is of paramount importance for many diseases.

To comprehend this concept, we must embark on a journey through our body's own metabolic pathways, reminiscent of Huckleberry Finn's pursuit of hidden truths. To survive our bodies have the ability to convert alpha-linolenic acid (ALA) from plants, a type of Omega-3 found mostly in seeds, into the longer chain Omega-3 fatty acids, eicosapentaenoic acid (EPA) and docosahexaenoic acid (DHA). Yet, much like a cryptic code that only reveals partial information, this conversion process is far from efficient.

The rate at which our body converts ALA to EPA is relatively low, as unpredictable as the twist and turns in a mystery thriller. Conversion rates are very low and depend on a variety of factors such as age, sex, genetics, and dietary components [38].

Investigations into this metabolic pathway have shown a very low and variable conversion rate of ALA to EPA, comparable to the unpredictable nature of Huck's journey. Depending on factors as diverse as the travelers Huck meets along his journey, this conversion rate can range from nothing to 8%. Many times especially in the elderly, fatty acid tests reveal there is no more conversion to EPA and DHA possible.

Multiple studies have taken on the task of decoding this mystery, striving to elucidate the conversion rate of ALA to EPA. The outcomes, however, are as variable as the plotline in Martels' Life of Pi saga. In men, the conversion rate is as minimal as 0.2%, presenting a cryptic conundrum that rivals any historic challenge our nutrition path has taken us.

Interestingly, like a fascinating subplot that enriches a tale, the conversion rate tends to be higher in women than in men. This biological nuance adds another layer of complexity to our understanding of Omega-3, a plot twist that further underscores the importance of direct EPA and DHA intake. [39]

As we embark on this adventure of comprehending the protective prowess of Omega-3 against common ailments, we must approach it with the same audacious spirit as Watson and Crick when they presented us with DNA double helix. At the crux of our journey lies a significant understanding: To achieve optimum health benefits, the daily intake of 250-500 mg of EPA and DHA is recommended, and for specific medical conditions, the suggestion escalates to 2-4 grams per day.

Our expedition to grasp this concept feels much like Huck's river journey, as we navigate through the body's complex metabolic pathways. We learned that our body is equipped to convert alpha-linolenic acid (ALA) into the essential longer chain Omega-3 fatty acids, eicosapentaenoic acid (EPA) and docosahexaenoic acid (DHA). However, similar to a challenging river bend that Huck might encounter, this conversion process is fraught with inefficiencies. The fascinating turn of events, that women generally exhibit a higher conversion rate than men, probably has evolutionary reasons due to the extra challenge to sustain a pregnancy. This peculiar fact, adding another layer to our understanding of Omega-3, illuminates the importance of direct EPA and DHA intake.

Several research endeavors, such as those conducted by Burdge, Wootton, Plourde, and Cunnane, have mapped out this metabolic territory much like Huck's navigation of the Mississippi. These studies consolidate the idea that dietary sources of EPA and DHA are more effective in raising their bodily levels than relying on the conversion of ALA.

So, akin to Huck's spirit for curiosity, resilience, and a quest for knowledge— This multifaceted narrative around Omega-3 culminates in a profound revelation:

To optimize our Omega-3 levels, and consequently fortify our shield against common illnesses, the direct intake of EPA and DHA from animal sources is crucial. These longer-chain fatty acids offer benefits that are as potent and transformative as the secret knowledge sought in a Leonardo daVinci painting.

So, let us approach our health journey with the curiosity of a seasoned symbologist, seeking deeper understanding, questioning established norms, and embracing the wisdom that Omega-3, particularly EPA and DHA, offers us. This is an adventure as thrilling as deciphering an ancient code, and as rewarding as discovering a secret that can fortify our health, and ultimately, enrich our lives.

Cardiovascular Health

As we delve deeper into our tale, we find Huckleberry Finn embarking on yet another adventure along the Mississippi. Despite being self-reliant, he soon realizes that living on a raft and navigating the vast river requires not only wit and courage, but also physical strength and vitality. He begins to feel a change in his stamina, his energy waning as days roll by. It's apparent that his previous diet with the widow, haphazard and lacking in nutrition, filled with cheap oatmeal and potatoes, is inadequate for this demanding life of adventure.

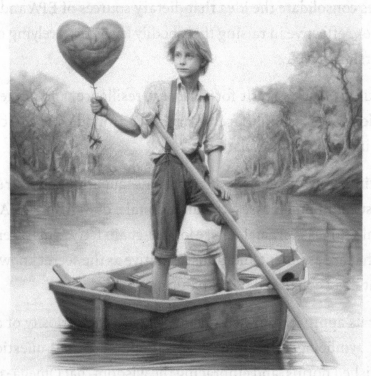

Fig. 13: Huck has a big strong heart

That's when Huck stumbles upon an unexpected boon. Along the banks of the mighty Mississippi, he sees locals angling for fish. Intrigued, he watches as they reel in their catch, fresh, gleaming fish that seem to embody the vigor of the river itself. Driven by his innate curiosity and his rumbling stomach, Huck decides to give it a try, and after numerous unsuccessful attempts and much laughter, Huck finally makes his first catch. He learns how to gut and prepare the fish over an open fire like it was ingrained in his memory. As he savors his meal, he realizes he's never tasted anything so delicious and fulfilling.

From then on, fresh fish becomes a staple of Huck's diet especially when he and Jim catch the biggest catfish ever. Over time, he notices a change in his energy levels. He's stronger, more agile, his endurance increased. No longer does he feel the fatigue of the previous days. He's healthier, his skin glowing under the sun, his eyes brighter. Huck feels an invigorating sense of vitality he's never known before.

What Huck doesn't know is that the fish from the Mississippi are rich in Omega-3 fatty acids, notably EPA and DHA. Consuming them regularly, Huck inadvertently stumbles upon the secret superfood that boosts his strength and vitality, helping him thrive on his adventurous journey.

Our story culminates with a healthy, robust Huckleberry Finn, the hero who, through his serendipitous discovery of Omega-3-rich fish, transforms his health and strengthens his ability to face the trials of his journey. Much like Huck's story, our quest for better health can lead us towards discovering the rich benefits of Omega-3, a testament to the importance of seeking out nature's bounty for our well-being.

Just as the Mississippi River is the lifeblood of Huckleberry Finn's story, so the heart is central to our own. It dictates the ebb and flow of our life story, every beat resonating with our body's tales of joy, sorrow, struggle, and triumph. Similar to Huck's reliance on the mighty river, the heart's function is influenced by the flow properties of our blood and our cellular metabolic processes. And just as the Mississippi river is full of twists and turns, so too are the factors that affect heart health.

Venturing into this complex territory, we stumble upon a precious ally: Omega-3 fatty acids. As pivotal to our journey as Huck's raft, Omega-3, in the form of EPA and DHA, can play a key role in enhancing heart health. Just as Huck adapted to the ever-changing river currents, our bodies can utilize these fatty acids to positively influence the heart's functioning. The European Food and Safety Agency (EFSA) echoes this belief, stating that a daily minimum intake of 250 mg of EPA and DHA can contribute to normal heart function. The reality is though that most of us are now far away from that reality.

Our adventure with Omega-3 draws parallels to Huck's journey of discovery and transformation. As he navigated the turbulent waters of the Mississippi, we steer our way through a sea of nutritional misinformation. Armed with knowledge, we begin to understand the profound impact Omega-3 can have on our heart health, and by extension, our overall well-being.

Just as Huck's raft carried him towards freedom, so too does our understanding of Omega-3 steer us towards improved health. It empowers us to challenge the restrictions imposed by a dietary landscape dominated by processed foods and misinformation. With each revelation, we gain strength, growing in confidence just as Huck did on his audacious journey.

As we chart our course towards a healthier lifestyle, Omega-3 is our constant companion, our ally in the quest for a healthier heart. As we further immerse ourselves in the vast world of nutrition, we carry with us the adventurous spirit of Huckleberry Finn, a reminder of the courage, resilience, and tenacity required to navigate our own health journey.

Just as Huck sought a world where he could live freely, we too aspire to a life where we are not merely surviving, but thriving. A life where our hearts beat strong, fueled by the beneficial power of Omega-3. In our story, much like Huck's, freedom and health are intertwined, each beat of our heart a testament to our continuous journey towards both.

Both DHA (docosahexaenoic acid) and EPA (eicosapentaenoic acid) are integrally involved in heart health in different aspects. Especially EPA may be particularly important for reducing inflammation, lowering triglycerides, improving blood pressure, and reducing the risk of arrhythmias, which are all important aspects of heart health.

Like a great river, the heart courses through our lives, silently and incessantly playing its tune. A healthy heart, just like the mighty Mississippi, promises us a robust journey through life. It's no coincidence that EPA, a potent form of Omega-3 fatty acids abundant in Huck's catch of the day, has been shown to be a formidable ally for the heart.

Think of EPA as a peace negotiator, quelling the flames of inflammation that can rage within our bodies, especially our arteries. As chronic inflammation is a notorious instigator of heart disease, EPA, with its potent anti-inflammatory properties, can be considered a sentinel, guarding our arteries against inflammation's corrosive effects.

Picture high levels of triglycerides like turbulent eddies threatening to capsize our boat. EPA, akin to a skilled navigator, reduces these hazardous levels in the blood, acting as a balancer in our turbulent lipid waters. This powerful Omega-3 fatty acid keeps our vessel steady, reducing the risk of us succumbing to the whirlpool of heart disease.

Imagine our blood pressure as the river's current. When it roars unchecked, it becomes a perilous force. However, EPA serves as a river dam, tempering the high blood pressure that otherwise could run rampant, eroding our body's landscape and contributing to heart disease.

The association between elevated triglycerides and heart disease is a widely accepted medical truth. Similar to how Huck used to navigate the treacherous eddies in the Mississippi river, EPA—this pivotal form of Omega-3 fatty acids—deftly maneuvers our internal river of life.

Imagine high triglyceride levels as debris of non-functional broken rafts floating in the bloodstream. They pose a potential threat, akin to submerged logs or floating detritus, menacing our body's health vessel. High levels of triglycerides add stress to the heart, just as a river cluttered with obstacles would complicate Huck's journey down the Mississippi.

However, EPA acts like a river-cleaner, diligently picking up these high-triglyceride "logs," reducing their number, and clearing the path. EPA, from the fish that Huck routinely caught, has been scientifically proven to reduce triglyceride levels, especially in individuals who have levels that are higher than normal.

Like Huck, who used his knowledge of the river to navigate the hazards, we can use our understanding of EPA to navigate our internal rivers and protect our heart health. Armed with this knowledge, we can incorporate more Omega-3 fatty acids into our diet, ensuring that we equip our bodies to maintain healthy triglyceride levels, thus reducing the risk of heart disease.

EPA is a powerful ally, a vigilant river-cleaner, in our body's river of life, as important for our journey towards health and vitality as Huck's quick thinking was for his journey down the Mississippi. By actively seeking to lower our triglyceride levels through Omega-3 supplementation, we are channeling Huck's cleverness and adaptability, setting ourselves up for a healthier, more vibrant journey through life.

EPA is also a master at restoring harmony when heart rhythms go awry, reducing the risk of life-threatening arrhythmias. It's like the steady hand on the tiller that keeps our heart's rhythm regular, avoiding treacherous cardiac rapids that can destabilize our journey.

Let's look at this in more detail. How then are the ropes of Omega-3 influencing cardiovascular disease by Improving endothelial function:

Consider the endothelium as the riverbed, silently supporting the life-giving flow above it. EPA works to keep the inner lining of our blood vessels healthy, thereby maintaining normal blood flow and warding off the dangerous encroachment of atherosclerosis. EPA's role in this context is like the diligent riverkeeper who ensures the riverbed is free of hazardous obstructions that could hinder the life-sustaining flow.

The story of Huck, EPA, and our heart unfolds into a vivid panorama of wellness, with EPA taking on a role akin to Huck's resourcefulness and perseverance. It becomes evident that a sufficient supply of EPA, either through diet or supplementation, is as crucial for our cardiovascular journey as Huck's resourcefulness was for his survival along the Mississippi River. Picture for a moment the banks of the Mississippi River, lined with sturdy trees and bushes that prevent erosion and maintain the flow of the river. In the realm of our bodies, this image is paralleled by the role of the endothelium, a thin membrane that lines the interior surface of our blood vessels. Just like those riverbanks, maintaining the integrity and function of this lining is crucial for smooth circulation and overall cardiovascular health.

Now, let's introduce our hero, Huck, in the form of EPA, one of the key Omega-3 fatty acids. EPA is like Huck when he's nurturing the natural environment around the Mississippi, tending to its health and wellbeing. EPA supports the health of the endothelium, enhancing its function and promoting its resilience.

The health of the endothelium is crucial because it orchestrates many complex functions in our blood vessels. It helps regulate blood clotting, immune responses, and controls the contraction and relaxation of the blood vessels, just as Huck would expertly navigate his raft down the Mississippi.

Through these actions, EPA reduces the likelihood of atherosclerosis, a condition where the arteries become clogged with fatty substances. This is equivalent to Huck clearing obstacles from the river's path, maintaining a clear course for the flow of the water.

In numerous studies [115, 116, 117], EPA has shown to improve the function of the endothelium, hence boosting the health of our circulatory system and reducing the risk of heart disease and therefore reducing other players such as triglycerides. Just as Huck's actions ensure the vitality of the river, EPA promotes a healthy, functional endothelium.

In conclusion, the power of EPA in the realm of cardiovascular health is as undeniable as Huck's competence in navigating the mighty Mississippi. This remarkable Omega-3 fatty acid not only fortifies the defenses of our cardiovascular system but actively works to keep it thriving, thereby shielding us from common heart diseases.

Mitochondrial health

Both EPA (eicosapentaenoic acid) and DHA (docosahexaenoic acid) are important for mitochondrial function and cytochrome c (the power plants and turbines of our heart muscles), but they may have different effects. The mighty mitochondria are much akin to the Jackson's Island in Huck's grand adventure. After Huck and Jim narrowly escape from their respective perils, they find refuge on this small, uninhabited island in the middle of the Mississippi River. It is here they rest, recover, and plan for the journey ahead, replenishing their energy and courage.

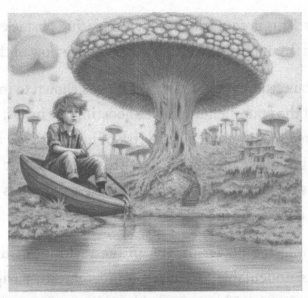

Fig. 14: Mitochondria are the powerhouses of our cells; Omega-3 is the instrumental component in the function of ATPase. ATPases are enzymes that break down ATP (adenosine triphosphate) into ADP (adenosine diphosphate), harnessing the energy released in this process to drive other cellular reactions.

Similarly, our cells turn to the mitochondria for rejuvenation. These tiny organelles provide a safe haven for cellular processes, producing the energy required for cell survival and function. They are the sanctuary within each cell where energy is created and stored for future use.

But just as Huck's stay on Jackson's Island was not permanent, neither is the energy produced by the mitochondria. Energy reserves become depleted, and like Huck, who needed to venture out again for food and supplies, our cells need a constant supply of the right nutrients, like Omega-3 fatty acids, to keep the mitochondrial engines running smoothly.

In this scenario, the Omega-3 fatty acids EPA and DHA become the sustenance our cells need. They are the fresh fish Huck catches in the Mississippi, the vital resources that keep the adventure going.

And when consumed in the right amounts, they ensure our cellular mitochondria – our very own Jackson's Islands – are well-equipped for the journey of life.

When speaking of EPA and DHA, the illustrious Omega-3 duo, it's essential to remember their roles extend well beyond the cardiovascular realm, delving deep into the smallest units of life – the cells. Like Huck and Jim relying on the raft to travel the Mississippi, each cell in our bodies depends on tiny structures called mitochondria, the 'powerhouses' of cells, producing the energy that cells require to function.

Our protagonist Huck, in the guise of EPA, emerges as an essential agent in this energy-production process. With EPA's influence, the mitochondria function more efficiently, producing energy at an optimized rate. In essence, EPA ensures the raft's paddles cut smoothly into the water, maintaining the raft's pace and direction despite the river's current.

DHA, too, has a role akin to a faithful companion, much like Jim in Huck's adventures. Like Jim's wise counsel aids their journey, DHA aids in increasing the functional levels of cytochrome c, a crucial player in the cellular energy generation process [118, 119]. It ensures the raft's design is sturdy and robust, capable of withstanding the river's occasional tumultuous currents.

However, the dynamic of EPA and DHA may parallel Huck and Jim's roles in their adventures more closely than initially appears. Huck, although young, often demonstrated an uncanny knack for making the right decisions in tough situations, just as EPA seems to have a slightly superior effect on enhancing mitochondrial function compared to DHA, according to some research. [120]

Despite this, just like Huck and Jim's relationship was built on a foundation of mutual respect and shared responsibilities, EPA and DHA work best together. They each contribute to the health of the mitochondria and, consequently, to the overall vitality of every cell in our bodies.

As we voyage into the mysteries of Omega-3, we find that just as Huck's story isn't simply about a river journey, the benefits of Omega-3 fatty acids aren't confined to any single facet of our health. These potent nutrients, like our intrepid adventurers, are capable of making profound impacts across a broad range of conditions and processes.

Let's imagine that, in the course of his journey down the Mississippi, Huck stumbles upon an old, dilapidated raft. It's barely holding together and seems unfit for the challenges of the powerful river. However, Huck, drawing upon his resourcefulness, reinforces the raft with sturdy branches, making it a reliable companion for his adventures.

The raft can be seen as a metaphor for our body's mitochondrial membrane, the 'powerhouses' of our cells. The energy is produced within the spaces of the double layer membrane. In a similar vein, Omega-3 fatty acids play the role of the sturdy branches that reinforce these cellular rafts.

Already the 1992 study by Benedict [40] metaphorically illustrates this dynamic, explaining that normal levels of these essential fatty acids in the mitochondria's phospholipids can rectify the dysfunctions observed when these fatty acids are deficient. In mitochondria isolated from hearts of dogs fed this Omega-3 rich diet for 60 weeks, the phospholipid content of inflammatory arachidonic acid was replaced by the Omega-3 fatty acids, eicosapentaenoic (EPA) and docosahexaenoic (DHA) acids.

The paper's revelations, in essence, describe how the deficient membranes, like a dilapidated raft, are restored to proper function by the Omega-3 fatty acids, thus ensuring the smooth 'sailing' of our cellular activities.

The journey of Huck Finn down the Mississippi is filled with dangers and challenges, much like the intricate workings of our bodies at the cellular level. And just as Huck depends on his resourcefulness and the strength of his raft to navigate these challenges, so do our cells depend on the critical roles of nutrients like Omega-3 fatty acids to maintain their health and functionality.

Therefore, ensuring a consistent intake of Omega-3 fatty acids is paramount to fortifying our cellular 'rafts', empowering them to face the tumultuous 'currents' of our daily lives, thereby safeguarding our overall health. As we further delve into the complex world of Omega-3 fatty acids, we realize that our journey towards understanding is as winding and enriching as Huck's own odyssey on the Mississippi.

Much like in the adventurous narrative we've been spinning, scientific research too has its share of unexpected revelations. Many studies now uncover how the proper function of cardiolipin relies on EPA and DHA. When the mitochondria have no access to proper Omega-3 the cytochrome c energy motors in mitochondria die. [124, 125]

Similar to how certain actions Huck took on his journey had different outcomes, the intake of EPA and DHA, both crucial Omega-3 fatty acids, influenced the health of our cellular Jackson's Islands

—the mitochondria - in unique ways. According to the study, EPA emerged as the hero, bolstering mitochondrial function and ramping up levels of cytochrome c in the skeletal muscle cells of older adults. These actions are akin to Huck reinforcing their island hideout and stockpiling resources for their survival.

On the other hand, DHA, much like a tool in Huck's inventory that didn't serve an immediate purpose, showed no effect on mitochondrial function in this context. However, just as every element in Huck's journey had its place and time, DHA too has been recognized in other studies for its crucial role in brain function and vision, solidifying its standing as a vital nutrient for our well-being.

In the grand narrative of our health, these findings underscore the need for a comprehensive understanding of the roles that different nutrients play and their distinct impacts on our cellular physiology. Just as Huck wouldn't rely solely on fishing to survive, we too must ensure a diverse and balanced intake of essential nutrients to support the myriad functions of our bodies.

As if we didn't know the centuries old truth about the importance of animal fat we needed science to reinvent the wheel. Once again Benedict 1992 [126] shows: Normal levels of the essential fatty acids in the n-3-enriched mitochondrial membrane phospholipids appear to eliminate the mitochondrial dysfunction observed in essential fatty acid-deficient membranes.

Heart Failure

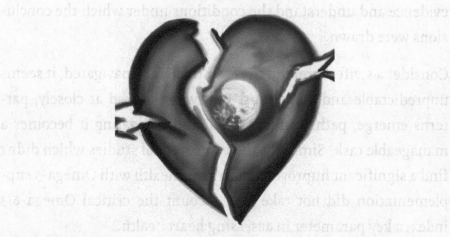

Fig. 15: Heart failure risk is directly related to Omega-3 and fish consumption. [110]

Arguably the most important health benefits you can get from Omega-3 supplementation is improving your heart health as we already discussed. Volumes and decades of research and clinical studies show the benefits of Omega-3. To be fair, there are meta-analyses studies that do not show any improved mortality with Omega-3 supplementation. How can that be? Scientists agree these studies are done with poor and inadequate supply of Omega-3 [80]. Omega-3 is a very fragile molecule and prone to oxidation, whereas Omega-6 is much more stable. This lies in the nature of the last carbon double bond (namely Omega-3) being easier attacked by oxygen.

But once you look at the Omega-6/3 index, there is a near 100% correlation of disease and Omega-3: the lower your Omega-6/3 index – the better your heart health.

In our journey to explore the true value of Omega-3, we face challenges not unlike those Huck encountered. While some might argue the benefits of Omega-3 for heart health, just as Huck encountered skeptics on his journey, we must look deeper into the evidence and understand the conditions under which the conclusions were drawn.

Consider a swift current in the river that Huck navigated, it seems unpredictable and dangerous. But, when looked at closely, patterns emerge, paths can be traced, and navigating it becomes a manageable task. Similarly, the controversial studies which didn't find a significant improvement in heart health with Omega-3 supplementation did not take into account the critical Omega-6/3 index, a key parameter in assessing heart health.

Like the Copernican Revolution, which shifted the world's perspective from an Earth-centric to a Sun-centric system, we need to shift our view of Omega-3 supplementation from a one-size-fits-all approach to one that takes individual Omega-6/3 indexes into account. It's about changing our perspective to recognize that Omega-3 supplementation is not a mere add-on, but a necessary balance to our modern diets.

Through this lens, we begin to see a more holistic picture. Similar to how Huck would observe and understand his environment to make informed decisions, we too should take into account the whole landscape of our nutritional intake. Understanding that the modern diet is often dominated by Omega-6 and lacks Omega-3, we can see how important it is to supplement Omega-3 to balance the scale.

As the sun sets over the Mississippi, coloring the river with shades of golden hues, we reflect on this journey of understanding Omega-3. In the same manner that Huck made sense of his world through observation and critical thinking, we too begin to see how vital

Omega-3 supplementation is for our heart health, not as a miracle cure, but as a balancing force against the flood of Omega-6 in our diets.

Let us take this lesson from Huck, to not shy away from shifting perspectives and challenging the status quo. For as we push past the swirling currents of conflicting information, we can better navigate towards the shore of better heart health and longevity. Just like Huck, we've embarked on an adventure that may just change the way we understand the world, in this case, the world of nutrition and heart health.

As we continue our journey with Huck, let's take a detour down a scientific tributary, exploring an intriguing discovery from 2009 that echoes the spirit of Copernicus. Just as Copernicus revolutionized our understanding of the cosmos, scientists Schacky and his colleagues shifted our perception of Omega-3 fatty acids. [41]

Imagine standing with Huck on the raft, scanning the vast river before us. The river represents our body, and the many currents and eddies are the complex systems within. One such current is the Omega-3 index, which Schacky [41] and his team studied extensively. They found that an Omega-3 index less than 4% was associated with a tenfold higher risk of heart disease compared to an index higher than 8%.

Consider how Huck would contemplate the river's flow, noticing how it changes and influences everything around it. The Omega-3 index, akin to the river's current, is a critical factor affecting our health's landscape, particularly our heart health. EPA and DHA, key Omega-3 fatty acids, are like hidden sandbars in the river, acting as antiarrhythmic and anti-atherosclerotic agents, helping to keep our journey smooth and reducing our risk of sudden cardiac events and non-fatal cardiovascular incidents.

Much like the way Huck would have to understand the river's flow to navigate it safely, we too need to understand the importance of maintaining a high Omega-3 index. In essence, it's not merely about supplementing with Omega-3, but achieving a beneficial balance between Omega-3 and Omega-6 fatty acids in our diet.

The lessons we draw from Huck's riverine adventures and Schacky's groundbreaking research are compelling. Like Huck, we must become keen observers, ready to challenge established notions, and like Copernicus, we should strive to change our perspectives, to reach a more profound understanding of the mechanisms that govern our health and wellbeing. As we journey onward, let us remember to seek balance in all things, particularly in our Omega-3 index, to keep the river of our health flowing smoothly.

Atrial Fibrillation (AFib)

As we delve deeper into the cosmic fabric of Omega-3 fatty acids, we find ourselves in the heart's rhythm section, the atria, where these essential nutrients demonstrate their skill as conductors, orchestrating a symphony that staves off the chaotic rhythm known as atrial fibrillation, or AFib. The rhythm section of the heart is as critical as the mighty Mississippi's currents were for Huck's raft —the difference between a smooth journey and a tumultuous one.

In the style of the intrepid Copernicus, researchers have dared to challenge prevailing notions and have illuminated a celestial body of evidence suggesting a higher Omega-3 index, much like Lemaitre and his team did in 2004. [99]

They unveiled that higher fish consumption, a rich source of Omega-3 fatty acids, was associated with a reduced risk of incident atrial fibrillation in older adults. A review from 2004, published in the journal Circulation [42], serves as a beacon, guiding us towards understanding how the essential harmony of our heart's rhythm can be maintained.

Think of Omega-3 fatty acids as Huck's reliable compass or Copernicus's astrolabe, guiding us through the vast, often perplexing landscape of nutritional science. They ensure our heart maintains its rhythm amidst the ever-changing tides of our body's nutritional needs.

Indeed, AFib is akin to a treacherous storm on the Mississippi, threatening to capsize Huck's raft. Yet, with Omega-3 as our faithful navigator, we can confidently traverse these potentially hazardous waters. By harnessing the protective power of Omega-3 fatty acids, we can maintain our heart's rhythm and significantly diminish the risk of AFib, reinforcing the vital role these nutrients play in our overall cardiovascular health.

This revelation, akin to Copernicus's heliocentric model, requires us to reorient our perspective, to acknowledge the importance of Omega-3 fatty acids in our diet, and to place them at the center of our nutritional universe. As we continue this journey, we come to understand the remarkable influence Omega-3 fatty acids wield over our health and well-being.

We must remember that not all fish are created equal. As Mozaffarian [99, 128] demonstrated in 2003 and 2004 "Persons consuming fatty fish twice per week had a 47% lower risk of coronary death compared with those who consumed fatty fish less than once per month", the preparation of the fish plays a critical role in its nutritional value and impact on health outcomes. Much like the deceptive calm of the Mississippi could swiftly morph into a deadly whirlpool, the nutritional value of fish can be drastically altered by frying.

When we fry fish, we are not only adding unhealthy fats but also causing changes that affect the Omega-6/3 index, increasing the ratio unfavorably. This shift reflects the precarious situation that Tom and Huck found themselves in when navigating the tumultuous Mississippi river. Too much Omega-6, like an unforeseen whirlpool, can send our health spiraling downwards.

Our understanding of nutrition has evolved, much like how Huck's journey opened his eyes to the realities and complexities of the world around him. We now know that the balance of nutrients, particularly the Omega-6/3 ratio, is of paramount importance.

Indeed, for arrhythmic problems, evidence is accumulating to support the role of Omega-3 PUFA as part of both acute and long-term treatment. This, along with mitochondria-targeted antioxidants, provides us with a new direction to improve cardiac health and decrease the risk of arrhythmias.

As we continue our exploration into the world of Omega-3 fatty acids, we come to appreciate more and more how integral they are to our overall health. Much like the river guided Huck and Jim on their journey, so too does the science of Omega-3 fatty acids guide us towards a healthier future.

Hypertension with Emphasis on Kidney Health

Indeed, the relationship between cardiovascular disease, hypertension, atherosclerosis, and heart disease is complex and multifactorial but may not be a mystery after all. This interconnected web, much like the winding path of Huck's journey on the Mississippi, is influenced by myriad factors, including our nutritional choices.

Omega-3 fatty acids, particularly EPA and DHA found in fatty fish or fish oil, have garnered significant attention for their cardiovascular benefits. These include their potential to reduce blood pressure and thereby mitigate the risk of cardiovascular disease, stroke, coronary artery disease, and hypertension-induced organ damage. [121]

Akin to the comforting, guiding light of the lighthouse in the midst of a stormy river, Omega-3 fatty acids offer a beacon of hope in the turbulent waters of cardiovascular disease. The American Heart Association, recognizing the significance of these fatty acids, recommends their regular consumption for both healthy adults and patients with coronary heart disease. There is probably nothing more important than keeping your kidneys healthy. All other organs have significant regenerative capabilities but the kidney is so highly specialized that once it is damaged the situation becomes life threatening and dialysis or an organ transplant is required. Chronic hypertension and toxicity destroys the delicate small capillary functions of the kidney glomeruli responsible for essential blood filtration. Without proper kidney function, waste and toxins can build up in the blood, leading to a host of health issues. These issues can include electrolyte imbalances, fluid imbalances, and the accumulation of waste products like urea and creatinine.

Over time, if not treated, kidney disease can lead to kidney failure, which is life-threatening and may necessitate dialysis or a kidney transplant.

Furthermore, kidneys also play other important roles in maintaining health. They regulate the body's fluid levels, balance the concentration of minerals like sodium, potassium, and calcium, produce hormones that regulate blood pressure, make red blood cells, and maintain bone health. Hence, compromised kidney function can impact all these areas, affecting the overall health and wellbeing of an individual.

The link between diet, particularly Omega-3 intake, and kidney health is complex and still under research. Many studies suggest that a diet rich in Omega-3 fatty acids has beneficial effects on kidney function. Simply by reducing inflammation and decreasing blood pressure your kidneys will thank you over time.

Nevertheless, in certain conditions such as chronic kidney disease, it's essential to consult with a healthcare professional before making substantial dietary changes. Consuming high amounts of protein can affect kidney function due to an increase in intraglomerular pressure and excessive filtering activity in the glomeruli. If kidney function tests show significant glomerular damage, excessive protein intake can be harmful.

Glomeruli, the tiny filtering units in the kidneys that produce urine from blood, experience hyperfiltration when they're forced to work harder than normal, as is often the case in chronic kidney disease. However, Omega-3 fish oil supplements can provide the body with necessary nutrients without putting additional stress on the kidneys. Omega-3 assists in repairing the body's tiny capillary vascular systems, including the glomeruli.

The results of this study [43] by Ulu show that an Omega-3-rich diet lowered Angiotensin-II, increased blood pressure, increased renal levels of EPA and DHA epoxides, and reduced renal markers of inflammation. How does this work? Epoxy products (essentially, the Omega-3 double bond is becoming oxidized) from PUFAs produce local electrical signals that are synthesized or generated in and released from the vascular endothelium that hyperpolarize nearby smooth muscle cells. This causes these cells to relax and thereby lowers blood pressure. This mechanism is very important for a healthy kidney and not just a systemic blood pressure. In other words if there is no Omega-3 present a local hypertensive effect in the Kidney can permanently destroy the glomeruli. Glomeruli are very complex structures that require a healthy blood pressure. Stanton 2020: "Eating the Omega-3 enriched foods resulted in clinically relevant reductions in diastolic blood pressure" [44].

The Story of Inuit Eskimos and Heart Disease

The echoes of Huck's rebellious spirit and Copernican innovation resound in our exploration of modern nutritional science. In fact, it's like navigating the Mississippi; one must be vigilant of lurking dangers, of consuming excess Omega-6 fatty acids, akin to the river's treacherous undercurrents, leading to chronic inflammation and heart disease. This critical correlation was revealed in a comparative study between the Western diet and that of the Inuit Eskimos in Greenland.

The American landscape, much like the chaotic river Huck traversed, is saturated with foods high in Omega-6 fatty acids, owing largely to the ubiquity of processed foods and the prevalence of oils like corn, soybean, and sunflower in our diets. The average person consumes up to 15 tsp of inflammatory vegetable oil per day, mostly unknowingly [46]. That amount is equivalent to >300g of sunflower seeds. This is only the result of modern industrial processing. These oils are loaded with inflammatory Omega-6 (up to 60%) and contain almost no Omega-3. For example, canola oil contains a small but significant amount of Omega-3, however due to food processing and long shelf times, by the time it arrives in your kitchen the Omega-3 is largely oxidized and the oil contains mostly Omega-6 which is much more stable. This unbalanced ratio of Omega-6 to Omega-3 fatty acids — often exceeding 15:1 — serves as a silent instigator of chronic inflammation, acting as a dangerous whirlpool in our nutritional river that can pull us under and contribute significantly to heart disease.

Country/Region	Estimated Omega-6 in [%] of total calories	Estimated Heart Disease Risk
USA	**High** (ca. 7-8%)	High
Quebec Inuit	**Medium** (ca. 5-6%	Medium-High
Japan Ainu	**High** (ca. 4%)	Low
Greenland (Inuit population)	**High** (ca. 2%)	Very Low (traditional lifestyle)

Table: There is a direct linear relationship between heart disease and Omega-6 levels in Inuit Tribes. [45, 107, 108, 131]

Now, let us journey north to Greenland, where the Inuit Eskimos have long thrived on a diet that balances these essential fatty acids beautifully. Their daily fare, rich in fish, seal, and whale — all teeming with Omega-3 fatty acids — stands in stark contrast to the Western diet. It's akin to navigating a serene, steady stream compared to the tumultuous, hazard-ridden Mississippi. The incidence of heart disease among Inuit Eskimos is significantly lower than their Western counterparts, suggesting a protective effect afforded by their Omega-3 rich diet.

Brain Health and Dementia

You will see much more on the effects of Omega-3 on brain development in later chapters but let's imagine our intrepid Huckleberry Finn having a peculiar dream one night on the raft, drifting along the grand Mississippi. In this dream, he meets none other than the revolutionary Nicolaus Copernicus himself. It's a dream fueled by an adventurous spirit and a recently nourished brain, no doubt a result of his newfound diet rich in the local river fish.

Copernicus, just as in his Earthly life, is intent on presenting a new worldview, shaking the very foundations of what was deemed unquestionable. Only this time, his proposition isn't about the cosmos but the human brain, about its magnificent design and the wonders that lay within its folds and crevices.

"You see, Huck," Copernicus begins, "our brain, it's an awe-inspiring universe unto itself. It's composed of vast galaxies of neurons, connected by a network of synapses. And within these synapses, a staggering amount of DHA resides. Almost half of all lipids in this phospholipid bilayer of our brain's synapses consists of this molecule."

With each word from the sage, Huck's dream-painted skies come alive with images of the brain, neurons, and synapses, mirroring constellations of stars, planets, and cosmic connections. "Sixty percent of the brain," continues Copernicus, "is fat, and of that, sixty percent should be unsaturated. You've been feeding your brain well, Huck."

Studies spun as stars light up the dream sky, showing correlations between Omega-3 intake and improved brain function. "You've stumbled upon a great secret, Huck. These fish you've been eating are not just filling your stomach but also nourishing your mind. By taking in at least 250 mg of DHA daily, you're maintaining normal brain function."

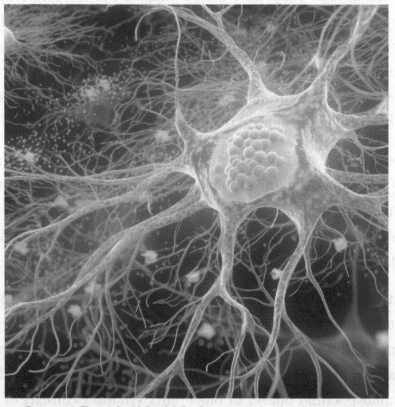

Fig. 16: Omega-3 Fatty Acid Lipid Rafts are involved in brain myelination (a layer around the nerve connections) and could revolutionize our understanding of brain development and aging. [47]

Researchers identified a special transporter protein, Mfsd2a (a lung cancer tumor suppressor gene, which regulates cell cycle progression and cell attachment), that plays a critical role in regulating the brain cells responsible for protecting nerves with myelin sheaths. Loss of myelin sheaths can occur during the normal aging process and in neurological diseases such as multiple sclerosis and Alzheimer's disease. Findings indicate Omega-3 lipids can direct oligodendrocyte development, a process that is critical for brain myelination [47].

And just as the sun begins to peek over the horizon, the dream starts to fade. But as Huck wakes, he is left with the vivid impression of Copernicus' words and the imprinted understanding of Omega-3's profound impact on the human brain. His journey isn't just one of exploration of the physical world anymore, but also an inward voyage of understanding the universe within.

"Huck, what is the most important tool for an adventurer?" Copernicus asked him one night. The dream had transported Huck to a serene riverbank under a sky full of stars. He pondered for a moment, looking at his trusty fishing rod lying beside him. "Why, I reckon that would be my eyes, sir. Can't navigate the Mississippi or spot a good fishin' spot without 'em."

Copernicus nodded approvingly. "Very true, Huck. Now, what if I told you that the very fish you catch can help keep your eyesight sharp?"

Huck looked at the spectral astronomer, intrigued. "Do go on, sir."

Copernicus, ever the patient teacher, elaborated. "The human eye contains a large amount of Omega-3 fatty acids. In particular, it houses a high concentration of DHA. This means that by catching and consuming fish from the river, you're not only feeding yourself but also providing your eyes with the nutrients they need to maintain their functionality."

As if on cue, the river began to shine, reflecting the cosmos above, turning into a river of stars. Huck watched as the glowing fish swam in it. "Now, imagine each of these fish as a source of DHA. Every catch, every meal, contributes to maintaining your vision. According to the European Food and Safety Agency, the positive effect is achieved with a daily intake of at least 250 mg of DHA."

Huck marveled at the starry river, the idea sinking in. As he woke from the dream, he looked at the morning sun reflecting on the Mississippi's surface, realizing he was not just catching his meals from the river, but also preserving his most critical tool for his adventures — his vision. Omega-3 was not just a nutrient, but a trusted ally, a guardian of his senses. With this newfound understanding, Huck was ready to face the day, eager for the adventures that awaited him. His journey wasn't just about freedom and exploration; it was also about discovery and learning — about the world, about life, and most importantly, about himself.

This comparison between dietary practices offers us an invaluable lesson. Like Huck, who learned to read the river's currents to keep his journey safe, we too must learn to balance our consumption of Omega-3 and Omega-6 fatty acids. Just as Copernicus dared to challenge the status quo, so too must we dare to adjust our dietary habits, to move toward a healthier balance, a more harmonious river of life. This shift, while challenging, is a vital step in steering our journey towards better health and longevity.

Omega-6/3 Imbalance and Cancer

There is increasing evidence suggesting that inflammation plays a significant role in cancer development and progression. Chronic inflammation can lead to DNA damage, which in turn may lead to the formation of cancerous cells. [48, 49]

Marine Omega-3 fatty acids, including eicosapentaenoic acid (EPA) and docosahexaenoic acid (DHA), have been shown to have potent anti-inflammatory effects. These fats, found primarily in fish and seafood, can help reduce the production of molecules and substances linked to inflammation, such as inflammatory eicosanoids and cytokines. Particularly colon cancer responds well to Omega-3 [51].

For example in breast cancer, some epidemiologic studies have found an association between higher intake or blood levels of EPA and DHA and reduced risk of breast cancer [50]. Again when it comes to clinical studies on Omega-3 and fish consumption results can be inconsistent, with other studies finding no association. These discrepancies may be due to factors such as differences in dietary assessment methods, differences in the types of fish consumed (and therefore the types of Omega-3 fatty acids), and the status of rancid supplements. However, researchers agree, when assessing the Omega-6/3 index the picture becomes clear that inadequate supplementation fails to reach therapeutically effective concentrations [91].

In preclinical studies (i.e., lab studies not done in humans), EPA and DHA have been shown to inhibit breast tumor growth, delay progression, and enhance the effects of some chemotherapy drugs.

How much more research do we really need to fully understand the relationship between Omega-3 fatty acids and cancer risk? Maintaining a diet rich in Omega-3 as part of a balanced, nutrient-rich diet, is generally recommended and established for overall health. Does this not apply to your cancer risk as well? As you can certainly discuss personal health concerns and dietary changes with a healthcare provider, keep in mind that blood tests show that most 'prescribed' supplements are shown to be ineffective and rancid. Your 'healthcare provider' should perform inflammatory Omega-3 index tests on a regular basis, to show that your supplements are working properly!

It's also important to note that while a healthy diet with supplementations of Omega-3 is likely to be crucial in reducing the risk of cancer, it is not a guarantee against cancer, and is only one component of a cancer prevention strategy.

It is important to note that while the Omega-6/3 ratio has a profound impact on health, it's not the sole determinant. A balanced and varied diet, regular exercise, sufficient rest, stress management, and timely healthcare are all pieces of the puzzle.

How does Omega-3 prevent cancer?

As discussed in the previous chapter 3.1 systemic Inflammation due to high Omega-6/3 ratios is at the root of destructive cellular processes. Apart from reducing inflammation research has indeed indicated that cancer cells may have altered lipid metabolism, which can include a deficiency in Omega-3 fatty acids. Omega-3 fatty acids, particularly eicosapentaenoic acid (EPA) and docosahexaenoic acid (DHA), are crucial components of cell membranes and have several biological functions that may inhibit cancer growth.

One of the proposed mechanisms by which Omega-3 fatty acids might inhibit the growth of cancer cells is by incorporating into cell membranes and altering their properties. This can affect the fluidity, flexibility, permeability, and the function of several membrane proteins and receptors. Changes in these properties may in turn impact signal transduction pathways, cell behavior, and ultimately, cancer progression.

Another possibility is that Omega-3 fatty acids are metabolized into bioactive derivatives (like resolvins, protectins, and maresins) that possess anti-inflammatory, pro-resolution, and tissue regenerative properties. These compounds might contribute to reducing inflammation, a key factor in the development and progression of many types of cancer.

In Summary, your ailments and controlling modern diseases such as metabolic syndrome and cancer rely heavily on a good supply of Omega-3. Just as Huck and Jim relied on their wits, the camaraderie, and a robust raft to navigate the treacherous river, we too must employ a multi-faceted approach to navigate the complexities of health and wellness. This includes keeping our Omega-6/3 ratio balanced, ensuring proper Omega-3 supplementation as needed, and following a comprehensive approach to health. This method of maintaining health and wellness entails maintaining a balanced Omega-6/3 ratio, ensuring appropriate Omega-3 supplementation as required, and pursuing a holistic approach to health. It is crucial to undergo regular annual blood tests, including tests for the inflammatory Omega-6/3 index and a full fatty acid panel, for this purpose. While the details of these tests are further explained in the appendix, it's important to note that these fatty acid tests should only be conducted on red blood cell (RBC) membranes, not just on the liquid portion of the blood.

3.3 How Omega-3 Keeps You Young

Now, Huck wasn't one to worry about age, after all, he was still a boy at heart. But the notion of staying young, of preserving his youthful curiosity and vitality, held a certain allure. The thought struck him during another one of his dream encounters with Copernicus, their celestial conferences serving as mind-expanding adventures on their own.

"Huck, imagine your brain as a lively city," Copernicus began, the stars of the dream-night sky arranging themselves into an intricate pattern that looked like a bustling metropolis. "Now think of Omega-3, specifically DHA, as the city's life force, the energy that keeps the lights glowing and the machines humming."

The star-made city sparkled brighter in response to Copernicus's words, making the point clearer for young Huck. "Without enough Omega-3, this city, your brain, would slowly darken, its buildings shrinking, its activities slowing down. In a sense, it ages faster, losing its vitality."

Huck watched the star-city shrink and dim, a sight that made his heart sink. But as if sensing his unease, Copernicus quickly reassured him. "But you've been doing the right thing, Huck. Eating fish rich in DHA is like sending a constant supply of energy to your city, keeping it lively, bright, and young."

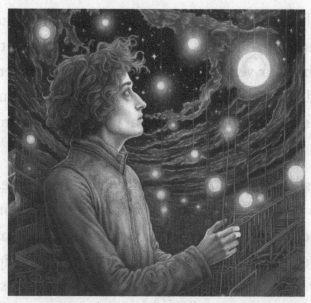

Fig. 17: As Copernicus changed our paradigm of the universe, Omega-3 revolutionizes the function of our brain.

Huck's dream city started to grow and glow again, now even brighter and grander than before. "See, with sufficient DHA, gray matter volumes in your brain are positively associated. This means you're keeping your brain youthful, vibrant, and primed for adventure."

As the dream started to fade with the approaching dawn, Huck was left with a profound appreciation of the fish he'd been eating. He was, in essence, feeding his mind's vitality, ensuring the machinery of his brain-city stays well-oiled and youthful. As he woke, he carried this understanding into his waking life, knowing that his Omega-3 rich diet wasn't just about his present health but also about preserving his youthful mind in the years to come.

As in the adventures of our young hero Huckleberry Finn, the river of life constantly flows, but as it meanders towards the sea, it inevitably slows. In our bodies, a similar journey takes place, a voyage marked by the ebbs and flows of life's energy, the vitality found within our very cells. Our cellular energy generators, the mitochondria, require the right fuel to maintain this energy flow. This fuel is none other than Omega-3 fatty acids, primarily EPA and DHA.

Now, let's step away from the riverbank and into the realm of the minuscule – the microscopic world of our cells. Within our cells exist strands of DNA, our genetic blueprints, that are capped with protective ends called telomeres, much like the plastic tips of shoelaces. As we age, these telomeres gradually wear down, shortening with each cellular division. When telomeres become too short, our cells lose their ability to function optimally, a process we experience as aging.

However, the tale does not end here. Like the secret treasure map in an adventure story, scientific studies have revealed that the path to longer telomeres and potentially prolonged vitality might lie in the consistent intake of Omega-3 fatty acids. As fascinating as the cryptic patterns on a map drawn by Mark Twain himself, the links between Omega-3 and telomere length are intriguing and compelling.

Talking about DNA, telomeres lengthen with Omega-3

Telomeres are the protective caps on the ends of our chromosomes that shorten as our cells divide. When the telomeres get too short, the cell can no longer divide and becomes inactive or dies. This process of telomere shortening is associated with aging, cancer, and a higher risk of death. Thus, strategies that might lengthen telomeres could potentially increase life span and health span. [52, 53]

Imagine, if you will, an enzyme called telomerase as a talented artist, meticulously working to restore the faded colors and details of a beloved masterpiece. Telomerase is the diligent restorer of our telomeres, the very tips of our DNA strands that wear away as we age. By increasing telomerase activity, we potentially extend the lifespan of our cells and our own vitality.

"Association of Marine Omega-3 Fatty Acid Levels With Telomeric Aging in Patients With Coronary Heart Disease" [54], a milestone study published in the Journal of the American Medical Association charted this unexpected course. The study found that among healthy older adults, higher intake of Omega-3 fatty acids was associated with longer telomeres. This research suggests that just as the river nourished and shaped Huckleberry Finn's journey, Omega-3 fatty acids may nourish and shape our cellular health, potentially extending the lifespan of our cells. Ali 2022 revealed : The results revealed an overall beneficial effect of Omega-3 fatty acids on the telomere length (mean difference = 0.16; 95% CI, 0.02, 0.30; p = 0.02).

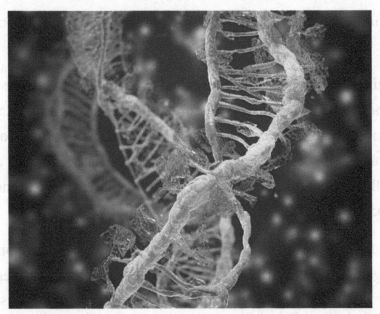

Fig. 18: Omega-3 affects the aging process through telomeres. [55]

Like Copernicus challenging the geocentric model of the cosmos, this idea challenges our traditional views of aging. Could it be possible that through Omega-3 intake, we have some control over the aging process? That we can impact our cellular vitality in such a profound way? The science suggests that yes, perhaps we can.

But just as Finn would not merely accept the word of others, neither should we. Each of us should set forth on our own personal journey, exploring how Omega-3 fatty acids can nourish our bodies and help us maintain our cellular vitality. This could be a game-changing revelation, transforming our approach to aging, just as Copernicus transformed our understanding of the cosmos. As we delve into this exciting frontier, let's remember the spirit of Huckleberry Finn, the audacity of Copernicus, and the pursuit of truth that unites them both.

The river of knowledge widens, offering new paths to explore. In this unfolding narrative, a 2014 study published in the journal

Brain, Behavior, and Immunity offers another significant milestone on the journey towards understanding the profound impact of Omega-3 fatty acids. Changes in the n-6:n-3 PUFA plasma ratios helped clarify the intervention's impact: telomere length increased with decreasing Omega-6/3 ratios. The data suggest that lower Omega-6/3 ratios can impact cell aging. [56]

Controlling Aging starts early in life: This study "Omega-3 supplementation lowers inflammation and anxiety in medical students: A randomized controlled trial" by Kiecolt-Glaser et al., published in Brain, Behavior, and Immunity in 2011. [56]

This study found that medical students who received Omega-3 supplements exhibited a reduction in inflammation and anxiety when compared to those who received placebo. The researchers also observed that changes in Omega-6 to Omega-3 ratios were associated with changes in telomere length, suggesting that Omega-3 supplementation may slow cellular aging.

A link between Omega-3 fatty acids, such as DHA (docosahexaenoic acid) and EPA (eicosapentaenoic acid), and ADHD (Attention Deficit Hyperactivity Disorder).

Multiple studies have shown that children and adolescents with ADHD tend to have lower levels of Omega-3 fatty acids compared to their peers. This has led some researchers to suggest that Omega-3 supplementation might help improve ADHD symptoms.

For example, a meta-analysis of many studies published in 2017 found that Omega-3 supplementation significantly improved clinical symptoms of ADHD. Furthermore, children and adolescents with ADHD have overall lower levels of DHA. [127]

They also reported that patients with ADHD had lower levels of EPA, DHA, and total Omega-3 in their blood, and that supplementation improved cognitive measures associated with attention.

The study by Alessandra da Silva [57] found that Omega-3 supplementation increased the activity of this cellular artist in patients with major depressive disorder. Here we see the subtle touch of our author's pen, connecting the intangible world of mental health with the physical world of cellular biology. As Huck navigated the difficult waters of personal and societal conflicts, the individuals in this study, too, battled the tumultuous waves of a major depressive disorder. However, it appears that Omega-3 could be a beacon of light in these stormy seas.

This study further supports the notion that Omega-3 fatty acids, akin to a life raft in the unpredictable currents of life, may serve to buoy our health and well-being, both physically and mentally. It hints at a deeper relationship between our mental health and the state of our cells, a link as intricate and intertwined as the plot twists in an engaging novel.

The potential of Omega-3 to boost both the longevity and the vitality of our cells is a proposition as audacious as the heliocentric model of Copernicus. Just as his revolutionary ideas caused a profound shift in our understanding of the cosmos, so too might these findings alter our approach to aging and mental health.

This trail of scientific revelations, much like the thread of a compelling narrative, invites us to question, explore, and venture into uncharted territories. It beckons us to be as inquisitive as Huck, as daring as Copernicus, and as open to new perspectives as the most riveted reader. After all, the story of our health is a living, evolving tale, one that we're writing with every meal, every decision, and every day.

Dementia starts early in life

Just as our wily protagonist Huck ages throughout his journey, maturing as he encounters the rigors and delights of life, so too does our body and brain. The aging process, however, isn't as discernible in our brain and sensory organs, much like the subtle growth and change in Huck's character throughout his narrative. This process of maturation, while often hidden from our view, is no less real or impactful. The words of Swanson, penned in 2012, resonate like an echo in the grand expanse of the Mississippi river, attesting to the profound influence of Omega-3 fatty acids on healthy aging. [58]

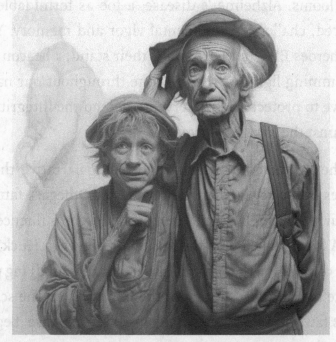

Fig. 19: Research shows that dementia in the elderly develops over decades of life. [58]

The development of a fetus, like the unwritten chapters of a nascent novel, is delicate and vital. The promise of tomorrow lies hidden within those first few cells, much as the seeds of a compelling narrative exist within the opening lines of a novel. EPA and DHA, the noble heroes of our Omega-3 narrative, play pivotal roles in fetal development, guiding the unfolding story of life, much like the unseen hands of an author.

With cardiovascular function acting as the steady rhythm of life's symphony, the influence of these fatty acids on our heart's health cannot be understated. They move with the precision of an orchestra conductor, directing the harmony of our body's workings. The heart, like the central plot of a novel, propels the story forward, its beat echoing the relentless passage of time.

In the twilight of our lives, as the pages of our novel near their end, a threat looms. Alzheimer's disease, a foe as formidable as any Huck faced, challenges our mental vigor and memory. Yet here too, the heroes EPA and DHA make their stand, a beacon of hope in the dimming light. As they've done throughout our narrative, they strive to protect and preserve, to defend the integrity of our story against the ravages of time and disease.

Akin to the pivotal moments in an enthralling narrative, these crucial stages of life reveal the true potency of Omega-3 fatty acids. As we journey through the pages of our lives, the influence of EPA and DHA is as pervasive as the Mississippi river in Huck's tale, a constant companion that shapes our health and our aging process. Much like the untamed waters of the mighty river, the science of Omega-3 fatty acids is a vast and compelling expanse, begging to be explored.

Your Stem cells matter

Much like Huck's youthful resourcefulness that maneuvered him through the turbulent currents of Mississippi, our body has a resourceful system – the stem cells, dynamic actors in the intricate theater of cellular regeneration. But even the most audacious protagonists require a nurturing environment to thrive. In the same vein, Rashid's insightful research in 2016 points out that polyunsaturated fatty acids (PUFAs) can serve as nurturing agents for our body's stem cells, akin to a calm river stretch that enables Huck to navigate his raft more effectively. [59]

But what does this mean in our understanding of the complex drama of life, health, and longevity? Rashid's insight weaves another thread into the tapestry of this narrative. Just as Huck's adventure could be reshaped by the changing contours of the river, our cellular fate can be influenced by PUFA-based interventions, a promising possibility that bridges the divide between abstract science and tangible clinical applications.

And just as the river held a myriad of unseen creatures beneath its surface, our bodies host a bustling cellular ecosystem. Within this vibrant tableau, stem cells play a crucial role. They are akin to Huck, shaping their destiny through an unpredictable journey of proliferation and differentiation.

The magic of Rashid's perspective is its practicality. In our adventure towards health, we must traverse scientific revelations with the same discernment Huck applied in negotiating the twists and turns of Mississippi. It is an invitation to reconsider our nutritional choices, to influence the environment our stem cells inhabit, much like Huck's strategic decisions to safeguard his survival on the unpredictable river.

This new understanding, built on the firm scaffolding of research, illuminates a path that can make the seemingly insurmountable challenge of controlling stem cell fate an achievable goal. It is a potent reminder that everyone is an active agent in the unfolding of our own narrative. And as we continue to navigate this complex labyrinth of health and longevity, the insights gleaned from the scientific frontier of Omega-3 testing, can guide us towards a vibrant and empowered existence.

A study conducted by Kang and colleagues in 2014 [60], which posits that interventions based on polyunsaturated fatty acids (PUFAs) might be a promising approach to influence stem cell proliferation or differentiation for clinical applications.

Polyunsaturated fatty acids (PUFAs), including Omega-3 and Omega-6 fatty acids, have been shown to influence several biological processes, including inflammation, cellular signaling, and membrane fluidity. Additionally, certain PUFAs have been shown to play a role in the regulation of stem cell differentiation and proliferation.

In this context, the researchers hypothesized that PUFA-based interventions could be developed to control the fate of stem cells, potentially aiding in the development of new therapies for diseases that involve stem cell dysfunction or for conditions that could be treated with stem cell therapies. [61]

Sarcopenia in aging adults

As Huck's strength and agility helped him steer the precarious raft, navigating the wild Mississippi, so too does our body require strength. Yet as we age, much like a once sturdy raft weathering through time and elements, our muscular strength wanes. This natural process, known as sarcopenia, has been a daunting challenge in the landscape of aging. Yet, the resourcefulness of science, much like Huck's inventive mind, has offered promising solutions.

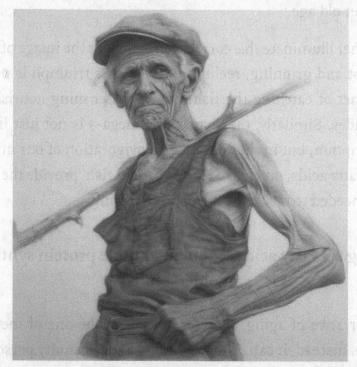

Fig. 20: Sarcopenia (muscle loss) at older age is related to Omega-3 deficiency.

One such solution takes inspiration from the natural world, much like Huck, who used the resources offered by the river and its banks. Omega-3 fatty acids, abundant in fish that Huck might have caught from the river, have shown promising potential in counteracting the effects of sarcopenia. Indeed, much like the dietary rewards reaped from a successful fishing venture, Omega-3 supplementation can augment muscle protein synthesis rates in aging adults, according to a compelling study.

In this intriguing scientific expedition, the humble Omega-3 stands as a beacon of hope, akin to the lantern Huck might have lit in the enveloping darkness of the night. And much like Huck's resilience, this nutrient, derived from the heart of nature, helps our bodies persevere against the onslaught of time, bolstering our strength, reinforcing our vitality, and lighting our path towards a healthier old age.

To further illuminate this correlation, consider the image of Huck, barefoot and grinning, reeling in a fish. His triumph is not just in the act of catching the fish, but in the ensuing nourishment it provides. Similarly, the victory of Omega-3 is not just in their consumption, but in the subsequent invigoration of our muscles. These fatty acids, much like Huck's caught fish, provide the sustenance needed to tackle the adventure of aging.

Omega-3 fatty acids stimulate muscle protein synthesis in older adults!

The narrative of aging, therefore, need not be one of inevitable decline. Instead, it can echo the vitality and ingenuity personified in you. Aided by the beacon of Omega-3, we too can navigate the river of time, strength maintained, ready to tackle the challenges that may come our way. Much like the tale of Huckleberry Finn, the story of our health and longevity, too, can be one of empowerment and resilience. Huck certainly was young but he also had very good fish Omega-3 available to him to pull through those perilous adventures. [62]

Much like Huck's raft was guided by the ever-changing currents of the Mississippi, so are the lipid rafts creating fluctuating forces of our dietary choices. Huck, in his youthful wisdom, inherently understood the bounty offered by the river was more than just a means of survival; it was, in essence, a source of vitality. The fish he caught not only filled his stomach, but also, unbeknownst to him, fortified his body with precious Omega-3 fatty acids, adding to his youthful vigor and resilience.

In a sense, Huck's adventures can be seen as a metaphor for the journey of health and wellness. His readiness to face adversity, his resourcefulness, and his indomitable spirit are qualities that we too can embody in our quest for optimum health. And just like Huck, we have a faithful ally in Omega-3.

For Huck, the river was his provider, his protector, and his path. For us, Omega-3 can play a similar role - safeguarding our health, strengthening our body, and guiding us towards a state of well-being. As Huck had a steadfast trust in the river, so too can we rely on Omega-3 to navigate the ebbs and flows of our health journey.

The Mississippi, with its wealth of fish, endowed Huck with an advantage many of us might overlook. In each fish that he caught, he was inadvertently harvesting a potent source of Omega-3. And these fatty acids, much like the life lessons Huck learnt along his journey, contributed to his resilience and vitality.

Just as Huck was sustained by the river's offering, our bodies too thrive on the benefits of Omega-3. Indeed, it's as if nature, much like the enigmatic Mississippi, has offered us a potent shield in Omega-3 - a shield against the common maladies of our times. So, we ought to harness it, much like Huck did with the river, to propel our health and vitality forward.

Just as the river served as a backdrop to Huck's coming-of-age story, Omega-3 plays a crucial role in our health narrative. And as Huck's story reminds us, it's often the natural resources - the fish in the river, the Omega-3 in our diet - that are the most profound sources of strength and survival especially in older age. The health of our stem cells play a crucial role in this process.

When we look at the trials of Huckleberry Finn, a raft isn't the only common thread we find with Omega-3. It's clear to see that a force just as strong, just as steady, was working in the young boy's favor. Hauling fish after fish from the Mississippi, Huck was unwittingly gorging on a feast of Omega-3 polyunsaturated fatty acids, a kind of inflammaging antidote which, as Dupont's 2019 study shows, might be a countermeasure against sarcopenia, the age-related muscle wasting. [63]

Just as Huck fought off societal shackles, we are in a fight against the persistent chains of inflammation and insulin resistance that hold our health captive. There is a beacon of hope in this struggle - the very Omega-3 fatty acids that Huck unknowingly fed on. They hold the potential to break these bonds by their anabolic effect on our muscles and their ability to activate the mTOR signaling.

What if we, like Huck, could defy societal norms, instead of accepting age-related diseases as an inevitable curse? Dupont's study suggests that the inclusion of Omega-3 polyunsaturated fatty acids in our diet might be our Mississippi river, our way to navigate through the perilous waters of aging and chronic low-grade inflammation.

Huck's tenacity and resourcefulness saw him through various adversities. Similarly, it is our turn to utilize the resources nature has provided us in the form of Omega-3. Just as Huck didn't merely survive, but thrived, so too can we bolster our health, fend off inflammaging, and possibly delay or prevent the onset of sarcopenia.

As we delve further into the parallel between Huck's journey and our health odyssey, it becomes increasingly clear that the Omega-3 fatty acids abundant in Huck's river-caught diet might have played a significant role in his resilient spirit. It is with this newfound understanding that we can hopefully tap into the power of Omega-3 to shield us from common illnesses, thus underscoring the importance of Omega-3 in our health narrative.

Drawing inspiration from Huck's story, let's meet the adversities of aging with courage, determination, and a fishing rod - metaphorically speaking - in our hands. The 'inflammaging' and insulin resistance, the hidden adversaries within our bodies, don't stand a chance against the potent force of Omega-3, our very own Mississippi River, full of life-sustaining fish. For a more comprehensive and in detail discussion of many common diseases visit Omega-3health.us/science.

Chapter 4

Unleash Your Athletic Potential

As we discussed, healthy stem cells through Omega-3 are key not only to aging but also to athletic performance at any age. Omega-3 fatty acids, which include eicosapentaenoic acid (EPA) and docosahexaenoic acid (DHA), have been recognized for their beneficial effects on many aspects of health, including athletic performance and recovery. [122]

- Performance: Omega-3 fatty acids may help improve athletic performance by increasing muscle activation and reducing fatigue.

- Recovery: Omega-3 have anti-inflammatory properties which can help to speed up recovery time after intense exercise by reducing inflammation in the muscles.

- Muscle Growth: Omega-3 are believed to enhance muscle protein synthesis (the process that leads to muscle growth) and might help to increase muscle strength and function.

- Bone Health: Omega-3 might enhance bone formation, which is particularly important for athletes who engage in high-impact sports that can stress the skeletal system.

- Mental Health: Omega-3 also have a role in brain health, which can impact an athlete's motivation, mood, and stress response.

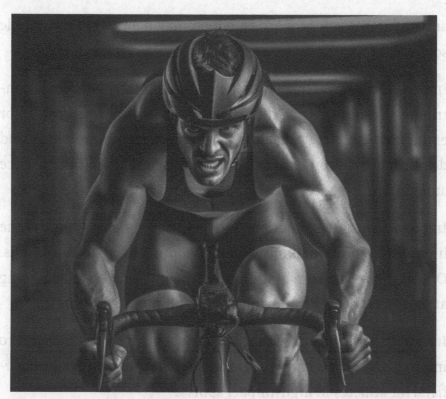

Fig. 21: Professional athletes, especially at older ages, are breaking new records when a reduction in Omega-6/3 index is achieved.

4.1 A Secret Fitness Companion

Omega-3 fatty acids, specifically EPA and DHA, may provide various benefits to athletic performance and recovery. Just as the steady and unfaltering flow of the river helped carry Huck and Jim on their journey, Omega-3 fatty acids might be considered a powerful ally for athletes. Here are some ways these essential fatty acids can potentially enhance athletic performance and recovery:

Reduced inflammation and muscle soreness: Exercise can induce inflammation and muscle damage, leading to muscle soreness and longer recovery times. Omega-3 fatty acids are known for their anti-inflammatory properties, which may help to reduce muscle soreness and speed up recovery.

Improved cardiovascular function: Omega-3 fatty acids may contribute to a healthier cardiovascular system, which is crucial for endurance athletes. A healthy heart can pump more blood and deliver more oxygen and nutrients to muscles, which can enhance athletic performance.

Improved immune function: Intense training can suppress the immune system, making athletes more prone to infections. Omega-3 fatty acids may strengthen the immune system, helping athletes to stay healthy during periods of intense training.

Improved joint health: Omega-3 fatty acids have been found to improve symptoms of joint pain and stiffness, which can be beneficial for athletes in high-impact sports.

Better brain health: DHA, a type of Omega-3 fatty acid, is vital for brain health and function. Improved cognitive function may enhance focus, decision-making, and reaction times in athletes.

It's important to note that while Omega-3 fatty acids may provide these benefits, they are not a substitute for a balanced diet, proper training, adequate rest, and medical advice.

Athletes put their bodies under significant stress through intense training and competition. The high metabolic demands of exercise, particularly endurance and high-intensity training, often increase the production of free radicals and inflammatory substances in the body. Omega-3 fatty acids, particularly DHA (docosahexaenoic acid), are known for their anti-inflammatory properties and can play a crucial role in managing and reducing inflammation.

However, given the high metabolic demands of athletic activities, athletes may require more Omega-3 fatty acids than non-athletes. If their dietary intake of these essential fats is insufficient, they could indeed become deficient, leading to an imbalance in the ratio of Omega-6 to Omega-3 fatty acids in their bodies.

A healthy ratio of Omega-6 to Omega-3 fatty acids is desired to be around 4:1 or lower. When this ratio becomes significantly higher, it can contribute to chronic inflammation, which may impair recovery and performance and increase the risk of injuries and illnesses.

Some athletes may show inflammatory index ratios as high as 100:1 due to their high Omega-6 intake from processed and fast foods and low Omega-3 intake, potentially leading to more inflammation and slower recovery times. This could highlight the importance of Omega-3 supplementation, a balanced diet rich in Omega-3 sources, and possibly personalized nutritional strategies for athletes to maintain a healthy Omega-6 to Omega-3 ratio and support their overall health and performance.

4.2 Fast-track Your Recovery with Omega-3

After weeks of their adventure on the Mississippi, Huck and Jim had grown accustomed to the rhythm of the river and the routine of their daily lives on the raft. They would fish in the river and cook their catch over an open fire on the raft. One day, they found themselves in the path of an enormous steamboat. They attempted to steer clear, but the steamboat was moving too quickly, and they ended up crashing into it. Their raft was destroyed, and they were left floating in the river.

Huck had always been a more enthusiastic fish eater than Jim. He loved the fresh fish from the river, while Jim preferred the cornmeal they had brought with them. The result of this was that Huck had been eating twice as much fish as Jim, providing him with a substantial amount of Omega-3 fatty acids, including EPA and DHA.

Omega-3 fatty acids, found in high quantities in fish, are known for their numerous health benefits. One of these benefits includes enhancing physical performance, which is exactly what Huck needed after the steamboat crash.

Despite the cold water and the strong currents, Huck found that he was able to swim with surprising strength and speed. His muscles felt energized, his movements were fluid, and he didn't tire as quickly as he thought he would. In fact, he found himself reaching the shore before Jim.

Jim, who had been eating less fish and thus receiving less Omega-3, struggled more in the water. He was slower and seemed to tire faster. He eventually made it to the shore, but he was exhausted and out of breath.

In the days that followed, Huck recovered faster, too. While Jim was still nursing sore muscles, Huck was already up and about, scavenging for materials to build a new raft.

Their experiences in the water and the difference in their recovery times made Huck and Jim realize the importance of a balanced diet. From then on, Jim started eating as much fish as Huck, ensuring that they both received the benefits of Omega-3 fatty acids.

While this is a fictional scenario, it illustrates the potential benefits of Omega-3 fatty acids, particularly EPA and DHA, on physical performance and recovery. It's important to remember, though, that Omega-3 maybe the magic bullet, and it works best as part of a balanced diet and healthy lifestyle.

Omega-3 fatty acids, including EPA and DHA, have shown promise in several areas that could benefit athletes or anyone undergoing physical exertion, like Huck and Jim on their raft:

Injury Reduction: The anti-inflammatory properties of Omega-3 may help reduce swelling and bruising following injury, accelerating recovery. This could be crucial in situations like the crash of Huck and Jim's raft, where rapid recovery might be necessary.

Muscle Preservation: Omega-3 have been shown to help counteract muscle loss and sarcopenia, the age-related loss of muscle mass and function. This is particularly important for aging athletes or individuals who want to maintain their strength and independence as they age. [123]

Reactive Oxygen Reduction: Physical exercise results in the production of reactive oxygen species (ROS), which can cause oxidative damage to cells. Omega-3 may help reduce the production of ROS, protecting the body from this oxidative damage.

Cortisol Regulation: Omega-3 may help regulate cortisol, the body's primary stress hormone. During periods of physical or mental stress, such as intense exercise or traumatic events, cortisol levels rise. By helping to regulate cortisol, Omega-3 could potentially help manage stress levels and improve recovery after physical exertion.

4.3 Real Stories

Super Athletes Who Love Omega-3

With many active individuals and particularly the elderly noting considerable improvements in stamina, strength, and endurance, it becomes clear that these benefits can be quantified through the performance metrics of elite athletes. Here, we'll share a collection of testimonials from both everyday fitness enthusiasts and professional athletes.

62-year old male

"I have only been taking the Zinzino balance oil for 6 weeks but this summer I was hiking on Mt Rainier and my wife was commenting me on how fast I was climbing up ahead of her. What were previously difficult hikes for me seemed much easier and I had almost no soreness in the following days."

57-year old cyclist

"I can now exercise without recovery time, I used be down for days with sore muscles and stiff tendons after a long ride. Since taking Zinzino balance oil for 18 month my heart is stronger than ever in my life. I feel rejuvenated and I can climb the steepest hills without significant heart pounding whereas before I had to stop and take a break, now I just keep going...- this Omega-3 product works well and gives me strength and endurance!"

A 22-years old Marine Soldier

"My fastest mile before taking Zinzino Balance oil was 6'30" about a year ago. I just ran 2.25 miles in 26 minutes and then directly went into another mile at a 6:30 minute pace and then directly into .75 mile at a

5:30 pace. Then a 1 minute break and I ran a 5th mile at 6:20 pace. I have been running more often than usual and I could have had a runners high from the 2.25miles at 10min mile pace (zone two I could hold a conversation during this) (and I had never gone into sprints after a slow run this long before)- I am more into my prime, I have more muscle etc although I weigh 60 pounds heavier now which could be a negative to running faster! In conclusion I think the balance oil is really good for athletic performance and had an effect on this test today. I had no fear for my heart when pushing myself, it didn't feel like my heart was pounding at all."

World Record ultra-cyclist, Arvis Sprude, setting several new Guinness World Records

"I hadn't paid much attention to my Omega-3 intake [64] before learning about Zinzino. I couldn't quite believe how bad my results were. My Omega-6:3 ratio was 17:1 and permeability of my cell membranes was 23.1. Now I understand that it's one of the reasons cyclists face various health conditions in ultra-competitions. [65]

One of the biggest indicators is my racing results. It's clear that ultra-cycling is an intense strain on the body, mind, and digestive system. I took ZinoBiotic+ everyday in the race I set the World Record. I don't suffer from digestive problems anymore. I feel like I'm only at the start of seeing what's possible with Zinzino = 2022: Team Arvis Arvis from Latvia cycled 2,211 miles or 3559 KM over 7 days averaging 315 miles per day or 508 KM per day. This beats the record we set in 2021 by 32 miles or 52 KM, cycling an extra 4 miles or 7 km per day."

A comment by Dr. Stuart Phillips, a leading researcher in the field of exercise physiology and nutrition. He's suggesting that Omega-3 fatty acids, such as EPA and DHA found in fish oil, might make skeletal muscle more receptive to the growth-promoting effects of resistance training and diet, thus enhancing muscle protein synthesis and helping maintain muscle mass.

This potential effect of Omega-3 could be particularly beneficial for athletes over 40. As we age, our bodies naturally start to lose muscle mass, a condition known as sarcopenia. However, by implementing resistance training and taking Omega-3 supplements, older athletes could counteract this effect, maintaining their muscle mass and strength, and potentially enhancing their performance.

In a nutshell, Omega-3 might help in preserving muscle mass, recovering from workouts, and reducing inflammation. That being said, there's ongoing research in this area, and we're still learning about the complete mechanisms and benefits of Omega-3 fatty acids in relation to exercise and muscle health.

It's also important to note that while Omega-3 can potentially support athletic performance and overall health, they should not replace a balanced diet and a well-rounded exercise regimen.

Omega-3 fatty acids like EPA and DHA are known to have multiple health benefits including reducing inflammation, improving heart health, and supporting brain function. On the other hand, while Omega-6 fatty acids are essential to our health, they are often consumed in excessive amounts in Western diets, which can contribute to inflammation if not balanced by adequate Omega-3 intake.

A high Omega-6 to Omega-3 ratio, as observed in many athletes and general population, can potentially lead to chronic inflammation and related health problems over time. By supplementing with Omega-3 fatty acids, the soccer players at LSK Norway were able to lower their Omega-6 to Omega-3 ratios, which could have potentially contributed to improved recovery, reduced inflammation, and overall better performance on the field.

Due to the high demand of tissue regeneration and energy usage Athletes have a higher cellular turnover. Building new muscle and the necessary vascular and neuro tissue requires large amounts of Omega-3. We see up to 95% deficiencies in tests resulting in inflammatory ratios of up to 100:1 in athletes.

Professional football players at LSK NORWAY were shown to have Omega-6/3 ratios in their blood averaging over 12:1, as high as 25:1. Only 2 players had an acceptable ratio below 4:1. After supplementation for 6 month the average was below 4:1. The club has since won the the Norwegian Football Cup and is currently positioned in the top third of the Eliteserien. [66]

So, how does this athletic miracle work?

Lactate dehydrogenase (LDH) is an enzyme that is involved in the process of anaerobic glycolysis, which is the breakdown of glucose for energy when oxygen levels are low, such as during intense physical activity. LDH catalyzes the conversion of pyruvate to lactate, a reaction that also converts NADH to NAD+. The replenishment of NAD+ is crucial for the continuation of glycolysis and ATP production.

Lactose Dehydrogenase Reduction Post Exercise

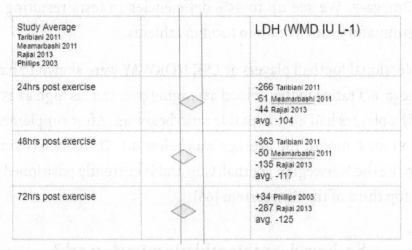

Study Average Taribiani 2011 Meamarbashi 2011 Rajiai 2013 Phillips 2003		LDH (WMD IU L-1)
24hrs post exercise		-266 Taribiani 2011 -61 Meamarbashi 2011 -44 Rajiai 2013 avg. -104
48hrs post exercise		-363 Taribiani 2011 -50 Meamarbashi 2011 -135 Rajiai 2013 avg. -117
72hrs post exercise		+34 Phillips 2003 -287 Rajiai 2013 avg. -125

Fig. 22: High levels of LDH in the blood following intense exercise typically indicate muscle damage, as LDH is released from damaged cells. Thus, athletes often aim to reduce LDH levels as a way of minimizing muscle damage and promoting recovery. Figure adapted from [67]

Some studies have found that Omega-3 supplementation can help to lower LDH levels. The suggested mechanism for this effect could be the anti-inflammatory properties of Omega-3 fatty acids, which may help to reduce muscle inflammation and damage during and after exercise. By reducing muscle damage, Omega-3 could potentially delay the onset of LDH release, allowing athletes to maintain high-intensity performance for a longer period of time.

Moreover, the anti-inflammatory effects of Omega-3 fatty acids could also enhance the recovery process, helping athletes to get back to training more quickly after intense exercise.

The importance of Omega-3 fatty acids, particularly DHA (docosahexaenoic acid), for mitochondrial health and function is very important. As mentioned, cardiolipin, a phospholipid found predominantly in the inner mitochondrial membrane, is particularly enriched with polyunsaturated fatty acids (PUFAs) such as DHA. Cardiolipin plays a crucial role in several mitochondrial processes, including energy production, apoptosis (programmed cell death), and mitochondrial fusion and fission.

Healthy cardiolipin composition is critical for maintaining optimal mitochondrial function. Changes in the fatty acid composition of cardiolipin, such as a reduction in DHA levels, can affect the fluidity and function of the mitochondrial membranes, potentially leading to mitochondrial dysfunction.

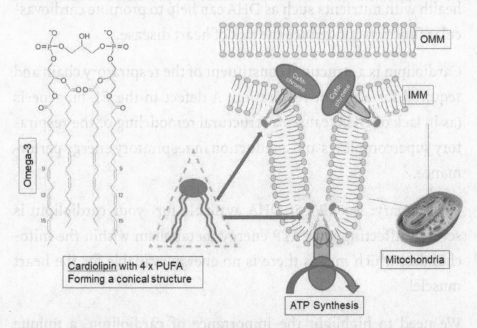

Energy Synthesis depends on Omega-3

Omega-3

Cardiolipin with 4 x PUFA
Forming a conical structure

OMM

IMM

Cyto-chrome

Cyto-chrome

Mitochondria

ATP Synthesis

Fig. 23: Cardiolipin, an essential component of energy synthesis in mitochondria, contains high amounts of DHA.

There is evidence [68] that DHA supplementation can promote cardiolipin synthesis and support mitochondrial health. In particular, DHA may help to preserve cardiolipin levels in conditions of oxidative stress, which can protect the mitochondria and support their function. Additionally, as a highly unsaturated fatty acid, DHA may influence the physical properties of the mitochondrial membranes, which can in turn affect the function of membrane-bound proteins such as cytochrome c. Research strongly suggests that when DHA oxidizes it renders the cytochrome c inactive and the mitochondria function will die. [118, 119]

On a cellular level, the mitochondrial health benefits of DHA can translate to numerous physiological benefits, including enhanced heart health. As the heart is a high-energy organ that relies heavily on mitochondria for ATP production, supporting mitochondrial health with nutrients such as DHA can help to promote cardiovascular function and reduce the risk of heart disease.

Cardiolipin is a structural constituent of the respiratory chain and required for efficient respiration. A defect in the CL-biogenesis (as in lack of DHA) causes a structural remodeling of the respiratory supercomplexes and a reduction in respiratory energy performance.

In summary: No EPA or DHA available for your cardiolipin is severely affecting your ATP energy metabolism within the mitochondria which means there is no energy available for the heart muscle!

We need to highlight the importance of cardiolipin, a unique phospholipid that is primarily found in the inner mitochondrial membrane, in supporting mitochondrial function. Cardiolipin plays a crucial role in maintaining the structure and function of the mitochondrial respiratory chain, which is the process by which cells generate energy in the form of ATP.

The fatty acid composition of cardiolipin, particularly its content of Omega-3 fatty acids such as DHA (docosahexaenoic acid), can significantly influence the function of the respiratory chain. DHA is a highly unsaturated fatty acid that contributes to the fluidity of the mitochondrial membranes, which can in turn affect the function of membrane-bound proteins involved in the respiratory chain, such as the complexes of the electron transport chain (ETC).

A deficiency in DHA can lead to alterations in the fatty acid composition of cardiolipin, potentially resulting in changes to the structure and function of the ETC and impairing cellular energy production. This could have significant implications for organs with high energy demands, such as the heart. Indeed, mitochondrial dysfunction and impaired energy production are key contributors to various heart conditions, including heart failure and ischemic heart disease.

Therefore, ensuring an adequate intake of Omega-3 fatty acids such as DHA, either through the diet or supplementation, is crucial for maintaining optimal mitochondrial function and supporting cardiovascular health.

In summary, Omega-3 fatty acids are incredibly important for overall health and particularly crucial in relation to athletic performance and recovery. Here's a brief summary of the benefits:

- Athletic performance: Omega-3 can help enhance athletic performance by improving muscle function and strength, boosting lung capacity and exercise endurance, and increasing fat metabolism.

- Heart health: They help reduce the risk of heart disease by decreasing triglycerides, lowering blood pressure, reducing blood clotting, decreasing stroke and heart failure risk, and reducing irregular heartbeats.

- Mental strength: Omega-3 fatty acids are essential for brain health. They help improve mood, increase focus and attention, support memory, and potentially delay cognitive decline as we age.

- Muscle recovery: They aid in post-exercise muscle recovery by reducing inflammation and soreness, promoting muscle synthesis, and speeding up recovery.

The inclusion of Omega-3 rich foods like fatty fish or supplementation (if needed) should be a consideration in anyone's diet, particularly those engaged in regular physical activity or high-performance sports.

Chapter 5

Boost Your Mood

The Yin and Yang of fat

5.1 Omega-3: Food for the Brain and Soul

Athletic performance and mental strength belong together. To understand this connection we are now addressing how Omega-3 is crucial in brain health in a short excursion into Traditional Chinese Medicine. What are its impacts on mood and emotional states? How does Omega-3 give you a better outlook on life and give you tools to make quicker and more efficient decisions?

Omega-3 fatty acids, particularly DHA and EPA, have a variety of benefits for brain health, which in turn impact mood, emotional states, and decision-making capabilities.

- Neuroprotection: DHA, which constitutes a large part of the brain's gray matter, provides a protective effect on neurons. This can impact cognitive abilities, including decision-making skills.

- Mood Regulation: Omega-3 fatty acids have been found to help in mood regulation. They are involved in the synthesis of neurotransmitters (like serotonin and dopamine) which are crucial for maintaining a positive mood. Low levels of these neurotransmitters are linked with conditions such as depression and anxiety.

- Anti-Inflammation: Omega-3 have potent anti-inflammatory properties. Since inflammation is now understood to play a role in a variety of mental health conditions, reducing inflammation can improve mental well-being.

- Stress Response: Some studies suggest that Omega-3 can help regulate the body's stress response, which is linked with mental health and decision-making capabilities.

- Brain Plasticity: Omega-3 fatty acids can influence the function and structure of membranes and thus help in promoting neuroplasticity, which is vital for learning and memory.

The Yin and Yang of Fatty molecules - An eastern look on how a healthy mind requires a healthy body.

The philosophy of Tai Ji 太極 (or Tai Chi) can help us understanding this connection. The 太極 is the ancient Chinese knowledge of the "supreme ultimate". It is based on the concept of yin and yang, the dualistic nature of reality, where two opposites coexist in harmony and continuously transform into one another. This philosophy also stresses the interdependence of the mind and body, as Yin 陰 can be seen as the physical form of the body and Yang 楊 as the formless spiritual mind.

In the context of health, this philosophy means that mental well-being and physical well-being are interconnected. Just as physical illnesses can lead to mental distress, mental illnesses can manifest as physical symptoms. Therefore, for overall wellness, it's important to take care of both your physical health (through a balanced diet, regular exercise, adequate sleep, etc.) and mental health (through stress management techniques, maintaining social connections, seeking professional help when needed, etc.).

Moreover, practices like Qi Gong, Tai Ji Quan, Yoga, Meditation, and other mindfulness-based exercises can help integrate mind and body wellness by promoting relaxation, improving concentration, increasing body awareness, and fostering a positive mental state. In these practices, mental focus, calmness and physical movements combine to achieve a state of mindfulness that can have positive effects on both physical and mental health.

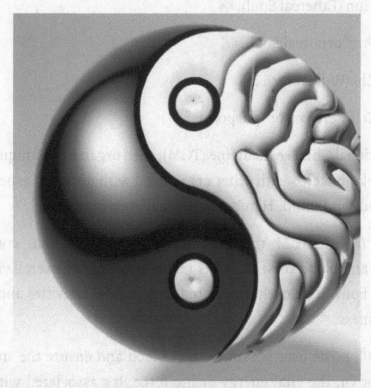

Fig. 24: According to the Yi Jing (易經 Book of Changes) and Traditional Chinese Medicine, the body and mind - yin and yang cannot exist without each other and they support and strengthen each other constantly.

Traditional Chinese Medicine (TCM) indeed has a different perspective on the body and its functions compared to Western medicine. The concept of the body in TCM is holistic and focuses more on the interconnectedness of different organs and systems. In TCM, the brain is indeed not considered the control center as it is in Western medicine. Instead, importance is placed on the main yin organs: heart, liver, lung, kidney, and spleen – as the centers of vital energy, or "Qi 氣".

Spirits are divided into [69]:

- Shen (Spirit): 神

- Hun (Ethereal Soul): 魂

- Po (Corporeal Soul): 魄

- Zhi (Will Power): 志

- Yi (intention" or "purpose): 意

Traditional Chinese Medicine (TCM), each organ has a unique role and relationships with other organs and with different aspects of the body and mind. Here's a simplified overview:

Heart (心): In TCM, the heart houses the mind (Shen), controls blood and blood vessels, and is responsible for the overall vitality of the body. It's closely associated with mental activities and consciousness.

Liver (肝): The liver is said to store blood and ensure the smooth flow of Qi, the vital energy or life force. It's associated with the Hun, the ethereal soul, which is responsible for planning and creativity.

Spleen (啤): The spleen is responsible for digestion and transformation of food into nutrients and Qi. It's associated with thought and concentration (Yi).

Lungs (肺): The lungs control Qi and respiration, and are responsible for forming a barrier against external harmful factors. They are associated with Po, the corporeal soul, which is linked to physical and sensory activities.

Kidneys (意): The kidneys store "Jing" or essence, govern birth, growth, reproduction, and development. They're associated with willpower (Zhi).

Each of these organs also has relationships with the others. For example, the liver and spleen have a mother-son relationship, where the liver (mother) can overact on the spleen (son) if it becomes too strong, and the spleen can insult the liver if it becomes overly weak. Such relationships are part of the Five Elements Theory, an important aspect of TCM.

Of course, this is a very simplified overview, and the relationships are much more complex in practice, involving other organs and elements as well. Understanding these relationships is a key part of diagnosis and treatment in TCM.

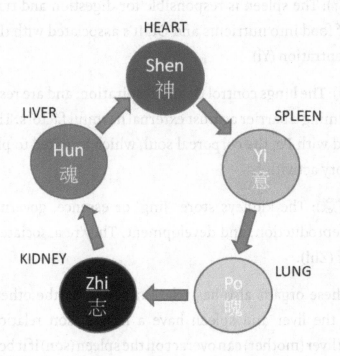

Fig. 25: Five spirits and their relationps to the five elements.

In more detail, Traditional Chinese Medicine (TCM) and philosophy, human consciousness and mental activity are understood as a complex interplay of five elements, often depicted hierarchically:

Shen (Spirit): 神 Shen is the highest element in this hierarchy, representing the human spirit in its entirety. It is considered the force behind activities and awareness, the essence that governs consciousness, emotions, thoughts, mental health, and life's purpose. It's viewed as the most 'yang' of the spirits. The heart, acting as the 'emperor' in TCM, rules the mind and the Shen, serving as the wellspring of wisdom and insight.

Hun (Ethereal Soul): hun 魂 Hun is closely related to Shen but represents the non-physical, ethereal aspects of consciousness. It is linked to dreaming, inspiration, aspirations, and creativity. Upon death, the Hun is believed to leave the body and merge back into the universal spiritual energy.

Po (Corporeal Soul): 魄 In contrast to Hun, the Po represents the corporeal, physical aspects of our existence. It is associated with sensations, physical reactions, and bodily functions. It's believed to return to the earth after death.

Zhi (Will Power): 志 Zhi represents the will power, determination, or drive within us. It is the element that fuels our perseverance and ability to achieve our goals. It's intimately connected with the water element and the Kidneys in TCM.

Yi (Intention or Purpose): 意 Yi, finally, represents our capacity for directed thought, focus, and intention. Yi houses the intellect and is responsible for logical thinking, analysis, and memory. It is connected with the Earth element and the Spleen in TCM. Yi enables us to concentrate, study, remember, and plan.

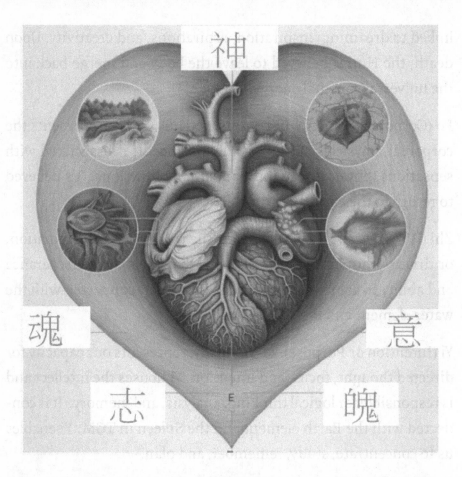

Fig. 26: The Heart shen 神 is believed closest to God and all other souls are subordinate and closer to the earth.

To sum this up, each Yin organ Heart, Lung, Kidney, Liver and Spleen in TCM is associated with a certain type of spirit and consciousness. This emphasizes the holistic perspective of TCM, which sees the body as an interconnected system where physical, emotional, and spiritual wellbeing are closely intertwined. However, this is a vastly different understanding from the Western medical model, which places a strong emphasis on the brain as the center of consciousness and control. However we do know that there is truth to this as the known phenomenon of transplant organ memory and the gut/brain axis. The phenomenon of "cellular memory" suggesting that memories, habits, and preferences can be stored in body cells, not just in the brain. This idea is sometimes proposed as an explanation for cases where organ recipients (like heart transplant patients) report changes in their tastes, behaviors, or emotions that they associate with their donor. Bruce Lipton's "Biology of Belief" [70] delivers a deep dive into this topic. That being said, it is true that the heart (along with the gut and other organs) has a complex network of neurons. The heart's neural network can function independently of the brain to some extent, which is why the heart can continue to beat even when it's disconnected from the brain, such as during a transplant. However, this is a far cry from the kind of complex neuronal processing needed to store memories or habits.

The gut-brain axis [71] is a term for the communication network that links your gut and brain. These two organs are connected both physically and biochemically in a number of different ways.

Physically, the gut and the brain are connected via the vagus nerve, the longest cranial nerve in the body. The vagus nerve acts as the "superhighway" for communication between the gut and the brain. [72]

Biochemically, the communication happens via the endocrine (hormonal) system, immune system, and the nervous system. For example, the gut microbiota (the billions of bacteria living in our gut) interact with the body and the brain through these systems.

This communication is bidirectional. Not only does the brain send signals to the gut, but the gut also sends signals to the brain. For example, bacteria in the gut help to break down food and in the process they produce various chemicals. These chemicals can influence the brain.

On the other hand, the brain can also influence the gut environment. Stress or depression can affect movement and contractions of the GI tract, make inflammation worse, or make you more susceptible to infection.

How do Fats play a role in this mind-body connection?

In Traditional Chinese Medicine, foods are often categorized as yin (cooling), yang (warming), or neutral, based on their effects on the body rather than their actual temperature. Yin foods are thought to help cool the body down, while yang foods are thought to warm it up.

Fats as food, being high in energy, are generally considered yang. They are thought to provide warmth and promote the function of the body's organs and tissues. This includes not just dietary saturated fats like those found in meat and dairy products, but also essential fatty acids like Omega-3. On the other hand, foods high in water content are considered more yin, as they help hydrate and cool down the body. These might include foods like fruits and vegetables, as well as certain dairy products like raw milk.

However, it's important to note that this classification is more nuanced than a simple division between yin and yang. Each food item has its own unique combination of characteristics and can have different effects depending on an individual's constitution, current health condition, and the way it's prepared.

A balance of Yin and Yang for optimal health

There is an integral relationship between lipid membranes and the functionality of each organ. We already established that life is essentially present in the lipid membrane and what that interaction between yin and yang means for the body. One could divide up the yin aspect of lipid Omega-3 fats as the physical membrane and the yang aspect to its "functionality" e.g. the inflammatory eicosanoids.

The connection between lipid membranes, specifically those rich in Omega-3 fatty acids, and the functionality of each organ in the body is fundamental. Every cell in our body has a membrane that is primarily composed of lipids, and the composition of these lipids has a major influence on the cell's function.

Omega-3 fatty acids, including DHA and EPA, are integral components of these cellular membranes. They maintain the fluidity of the cell membranes, which is essential for the cells' ability to function properly. For example, neurons in the brain need this fluidity to transmit signals efficiently. For that reason, the body stores little saturated fats (25% max relative to mono- and poly-unsaturated fats). [73]

In terms of the yin and yang philosophy, Omega-3 fatty acids could indeed be viewed as having both aspects. The physical presence of these fatty acids in the cell membrane (their structural role) could be considered the yin aspect: they provide structure and stability. The "yang" aspects could be seen as their dynamic role in cell signaling and inflammation, which involves their conversion into various eicosanoids, substances that have hormone-like effects and play a role in various bodily functions including the immune response.

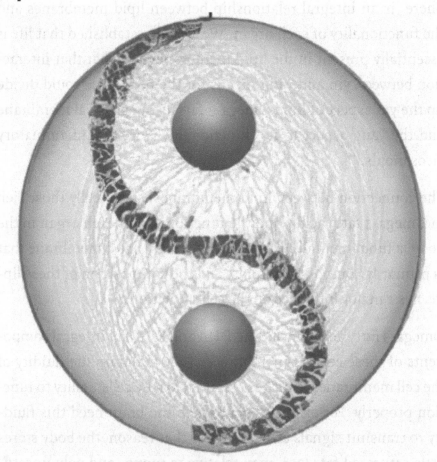

Fig. 27: Fat is both, Yin 陰 and Yang 楊

This global balance and interplay between structure (yin) and function (yang) is a key aspect of how Omega-3 fatty acids contribute to health. The inflammatory response (yang) is necessary for protecting the body and promoting healing, but it needs to be well-regulated and balanced by the structural stability (yin) to maintain health and prevent disease. Yin and yang are opposite energies that attract each other and together create a whole and balanced energy. When life-force energy is appropriately balanced between yin and yang, it flows smoothly maintaining and promoting a good state of physical and emotional health.

5.2 Feeling Blue? Omega-3 to the Rescue

As a reminder the brain consists of up to 60% of fat lipids. There's a growing body of evidence suggesting that Omega-3 fatty acids play a significant role in brain health and mood regulation. The two main types of Omega-3 fatty acids, eicosapentaenoic acid (EPA) and docosahexaenoic acid (DHA), are found in large amounts in the brain and are crucial for normal brain function. That is why the brain contains >12% of its relative mass in Omega-3. [74]

Your Brain shrinks without Omega-3

A study by Dr. William S. Harris and Dr. James V. Pottala, published in 2014, indeed reported a link between higher levels of Omega-3 fatty acids in the blood (specifically, the "Omega-3 index," which measures the amount of eicosapentaenoic acid (EPA) and docosahexaenoic acid (DHA) in red blood cell membranes) and larger brain volumes in older adults. [75]

The researchers analyzed data from 1,111 women who participated in the Women's Health Initiative Memory Study. They found that the women with higher Omega-3 index levels had larger total brain volumes and hippocampal volumes. The hippocampus is a region of the brain involved in memory and is often targeted in diseases like Alzheimer's.

Specifically, they found that a one-point increase in the Omega-3 index was associated with a 0.63% greater total brain volume, and a 2.7% greater hippocampal volume. This was measured over the course of 8-10 years.

Omega-3 prevents brain shrinkage (Pottala 2014)

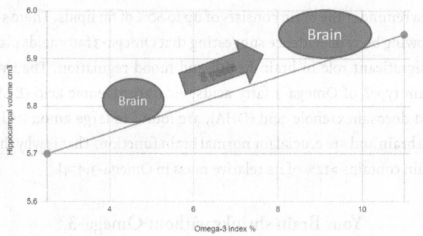

Fig. 28: Your brain grows with more Omega-3 intake. This figure is adapted from [75].

In simpler terms, the study showed a 3.2% greater Omega-3 index corresponded to a roughly 100 mm^3 larger hippocampal volume. The average natural level of EPA in the blood is recommended at 3.6%, while that of DHA is 4.7%, and combined they need to be above 8%, preferably 10%. The daily requirement of marine Omega-3 EPA and DHA depends on body type and demand. Eg. an athlete has a much higher demand on DHA. Over 90% of the population tests with indices of much below 4%. Adults weighing 80 kg need to consume approximately 3 grams of Omega-3 (EPA + DHA) daily to get their Omega-3 (EPA + DHA) level above 8%.

"A recent dose-response study found that 12 months of 0.93 and 1.86 g/d of EPA 1 DHA increased RBC levels by 3.6% and 4.5%, respectively. Therefore, changes in the Omega-3 index that can be achieved through diet modification and/or supplementation are similar to those associated with 1 to 2 years of normal, age-related brain atrophy." [76]

It is long known that dementia and brain shrinkage go along. In a previous study (2005) with 370 men and women followed over decades. Whole-brain volume differences were detected by age 30 and nondemented individuals had a mean decline of -0.45% per year but In those individuals with very mild DAT, the atrophy rate more than doubled (-0.98% per year) [77].

Another study from Chen (2020) shows: "For each interquartile increment (2.02%) in Omega-3 index, the average volume was 5.03 cm3 (p < 0.01) greater in the white matter and 0.08 cm3 (p = 0.03) greater in the hippocampus." The study shows how Omega-3 protects the brain from potential adverse effects of air pollution on white matter volumes [78].

How does the brain protection mechanism work?

EPA is involved in the biochemical pathway that produces eicosanoids, compounds that have various roles in the body's immune and inflammation responses. An imbalance in the body's levels of eicosanoids can result in inflammation and is thought to play a role in mental health disorders such as depression. Therefore, having adequate levels of EPA from sources like Omega-3 can help ensure a proper balance of eicosanoids, which in turn supports mood regulation and overall mental well-being.

DHA, on the other hand, is a major structural component of the brain and the retina of the eyes. It plays a vital role in the development and function of these organs, particularly in early life and during pregnancy. Once again, research shows that lipid membranes and their channels, pumps and receptors cannot be properly functional without DHA. The lipid rafts constitute the lifeline in your brain.

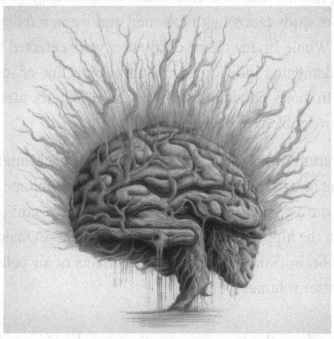

Fig. 29: Your brain is literally on fire from the excess inflammation produced by Omega-6 and the deficiency of Omega-3; this deficiency inhibits the neuronal function.

Notably, EPA and DHA are essential so your brain is in a constant inflammatory mode. Even if a non-rancid supply of alpha-linolenic acid (ALA) is present in your diet; EPA and DHA are not produced in large enough amounts by the human body, so they must be obtained from the diet or from supplements. As discussed, sources of EPA and DHA rich Omega-3 include fatty fish like salmon, herring and mackerel, or fish roe. Plant sources like flaxseeds, walnuts, and certain types of algae can only provide alpha-linolenic acid (ALA) on EPA or DHA.

A more recent meta-analyses from Dighriri 2022: "Omega-3 for brain performance In participants taking DHA supplements, serum DHA concentrations quadrupled and were associated with better PAL scores (paired associate learning; P<0.02)." DHA was well-tolerated and recorded with no major side effects study to found a positive association between the intake of DHA (docosahexaenoic acid), one of the key Omega-3 fatty acids, and improved scores on the Paired Associate Learning (PAL) test. The PAL test is a neuropsychological test often used to assess visual memory and new learning. Of 63 possible bias array assessments only 2 were identified as high risk.

This finding aligns with other research suggesting that DHA can support cognitive function and brain health. DHA is a major component of the gray matter of the brain and also of the retina in the eyes. It is crucial for the development of the nervous system as well as visual abilities in young infants. In adults, DHA seems to be important for maintenance of normal brain function.

This study from Satizabal [82] shows how of 2,183 dementia-free and stroke-free participants (mean age of 46 years, 53% women) a higher Omega-3 index was associated with larger hippocampal volumes and better abstract reasoning. Interestingly similar results were obtained for DHA or EPA concentrations individually. In addition the APOE-e4 status which is an indicator for Alzheimer's disease showed associations between higher DHA concentrations and larger hippocampal volumes in APOE-e4 noncarriers, whereas higher EPA concentrations were related to better abstract reasoning in positive APOE-e4 carriers. Finally, higher levels of all Omega-3 predictors were related to lower white matter hyperintensity burden (a stroke indicator) but only in APOE-e4 carriers.

Since 2004, the scientific community has adopted the Omega-6/3 index to analyze clinical studies properly! The relationship between this simple blood test marker and the risk for heart disease and dementia is very strong. [19]

In summary, ensuring sufficient intake of Omega-3 fatty acids can support overall brain health and mood regulation, likely due to their role in inflammation regulation and their structural importance in the brain. This inflammatory index can be measured before and after supplementation and diet changes. Studies show: It is imperative that the Omega-6/3 index moves below a ratio of 4:1! Depending on the starting index this process naturally can take up to 2 years. In other words, it takes longer from a starting ratio of 50:1 than it takes from 10:1 to get to the desired result. Ratios of 1.5:1 are possible after 3 or more years.

5.3 How Omega-3 Helps with Other Mental Disorders and Dementia

As briefly discussed in chapter 3.2, brain health is integrally linked to Omega-3. A very large percentage of the brain mass should consist of Omega-3 fatty acids. There is evidence suggesting that Omega-3 fatty acid deficiency early in life may be linked to an increased risk of developing mental health disorders. Omega-3 fatty acids, particularly docosahexaenoic acid (DHA) and eicosapentaenoic acid (EPA), are crucial for brain development and function throughout life.

Particularly docosahexaenoic acid (DHA), for brain development and mental health. Omega-3 fatty acids are critical for neurodevelopment during both prenatal and postnatal life. They are essential components of the brain and retina and play key roles in cell signaling, gene expression, and inflammation regulation.

Several studies suggest that early life Omega-3 deficiency can have long-lasting effects on cognitive development and mental health. These effects may include:

Cognitive Development: DHA is crucial for the development and function of the brain. A deficiency in Omega-3 during crucial developmental periods could potentially lead to cognitive delays or deficits.

Mental Health: Omega-3 are crucial for maintaining the structural and functional integrity of neuronal membranes, which is essential for effective neurotransmission. An imbalance in fatty acid composition could potentially contribute to mental health disorders such as depression, anxiety, and ADHD.

Neurodevelopmental Disorders: There is also some evidence suggesting that Omega-3 deficiency could contribute to the development of neurodevelopmental disorders such as autism and ADHD, although more research is needed in this area.

Dementia and Cognitive Decline: While the link between early life Omega-3 status and risk of dementia later in life is less clear, there is evidence that maintaining adequate Omega-3 intake throughout life may help protect against age-related cognitive decline and dementia.

Given the crucial role of Omega-3 fatty acids in brain health and development, ensuring adequate intake during pregnancy and early life is of paramount importance.

DHA is a major structural component of neuronal cell membranes and plays a vital role in maintaining their integrity and fluidity, while both DHA and EPA have anti-inflammatory and neuroprotective properties. As discussed, adequate Omega-3 fatty acid intake during critical periods of brain development, such as during pregnancy and early childhood, is essential for optimal cognitive and behavioral outcomes later in life.

Some of the mental health disorders potentially linked to Omega-3 deficiency early in life include:

Attention Deficit Hyperactivity Disorder (ADHD): Some studies have found that children with ADHD have lower levels of Omega-3 fatty acids, particularly DHA, compared to their peers. Omega-3 supplementation has shown potential benefits in improving ADHD symptoms in some clinical trials, although more research is needed to confirm these findings. [83]

Autism Spectrum Disorder (ASD): While the exact cause of ASD is not fully understood, some research has suggested that Omega-3 fatty acid deficiency during early brain development may be a contributing factor. Some studies have reported improvements in ASD symptoms following Omega-3 supplementation, but more research is necessary to establish a clear link.

Depression and anxiety: Omega-3 fatty acids have been shown to play a role in regulating mood and reducing inflammation, which can contribute to the development of depression and anxiety. Some studies have suggested that low Omega-3 levels during early life may be associated with an increased risk of developing these mental health disorders later in life. [84]

Schizophrenia and other psychotic disorders: There is some evidence suggesting that Omega-3 fatty acid deficiency during early brain development may increase the risk of developing schizophrenia and other psychotic disorders. Some studies have reported improvements in symptoms with Omega-3 supplementation. [85]

It is important to note that while Omega-3 deficiency may be a contributing factor to the development of mental health disorders, it is not the sole cause. Mental health disorders are complex and multifactorial, involving epigenetic, environmental, and lifestyle factors. However it is evident that Ensuring adequate Omega-3 intake during pregnancy and early childhood may be beneficial for promoting optimal brain development and reducing the risk of mental health disorders.

There is growing interest in the potential role of Omega-3 fatty acids in the prevention and management of Parkinson's disease (PD), a neurodegenerative disorder characterized by the progressive loss of dopaminergic neurons in the substantia nigra region of the brain. While the exact cause of PD is not yet fully understood, factors such as oxidative stress, inflammation, and mitochondrial dysfunction are believed to contribute to the development and progression of the disease especially in the area of lipid rafts. [86, 87]

Omega-3 fatty acids, particularly eicosapentaenoic acid (EPA) and docosahexaenoic acid (DHA), are known to have anti-inflammatory and neuroprotective properties, which could be beneficial in the context of Parkinson's disease. Some potential mechanisms by which Omega-3 fatty acids may influence PD include:

Reducing inflammation: Omega-3 fatty acids can modulate the production of inflammatory cytokines and other molecules involved in the inflammatory response, which could help protect dopaminergic neurons from damage associated with inflammation.

Protecting against oxidative stress: EPA and DHA have antioxidant properties and can help counteract the harmful effects of reactive oxygen species (ROS), which contribute to oxidative stress and neuronal damage in PD.

Supporting neuronal membrane integrity: DHA is a major structural component of neuronal cell membranes and plays a crucial role in maintaining their integrity and fluidity. Adequate DHA levels may support neuronal function and protect against neurodegeneration.

Promoting neurogenesis: Some studies have suggested that Omega-3 fatty acids could stimulate the growth of new neurons and support the survival of existing ones, which could be beneficial in slowing the progression of PD.

Evidence from preclinical studies and epidemiological research suggests that Omega-3 fatty acids may have protective effects against Parkinson's disease. Some data may not be conclusive due to the fact of inadequate supplements. Randomized controlled trials investigating the effects of proper Omega-3 supplementation in individuals with PD are necessary to establish the potential therapeutic benefits of these fatty acids in the prevention and management of the disease. However fish eaters show a clear benefit advantage when it comes to the risk of Parkinson's disease.

Several studies have examined the potential relationship between fish consumption and the risk of Parkinson's disease. Many cold water fish are high in Omega-3 fatty acids, which have been suggested to have neuroprotective effects and could potentially Lower the risk of Parkinson's disease. Additionally, fish is a significant source of dietary vitamin D, which has also been suggested to have a protective effect against Parkinson's.

It is important to get your Omega-3 from tested, small cold water fish to minimize the environmental toxins such as mercury, which could potentially increase the risk of neurodegenerative diseases such as Parkinson's.

A large Swedish study published in 2014 in the American Journal of Epidemiology found no overall association between fish consumption and depression in women [132]. These studies find a lower risk particularly among those who ate fatty fish and fish rich in Omega-3. Another study published in Neurology in 2020, suggested that even moderate consumption of dietary Omega-3 and vitamin D may be associated with a lower risk of Parkinson's disease. [133, 134]

Another study published in Neurology in 2003, suggested that even moderate consumption of dietary vitamin D may be associated with a lower risk of Parkinson's disease.

Particularly DHA is important in brain repair in all dementia diseases. What do the studies say:

Parkinson's and Alzheimer's studies show Indeed, treatment with Omega-3 fatty acids, being safe and well tolerated, represents a valuable and biologically plausible tool in the management of neurodegenerative diseases in their early stages. Most dementia diseases are age related. Our bodies are amazing designs that can operate on a level of below 10% optimal nutrition for a long time, however at a certain age and most Parkinson's is diagnosed above 65 years, the inflammation in the brain reaches a limit. A diet rich in Omega 3 can defeat the outcome of dementia! [88]

Parkinson's and lipid rafts

Evidence suggests the greatest benefit may be seen with DHA in non-cognitively impaired older people. Purified lipid rafts from the frontal cortex of postmortem samples from patients with early motor stage PD and incidental PD exhibit significant reductions in DHA (and AA), but not EPA or DPA, compared to controls (Fabelo et al., 2011). Dyall SC. Long-chain Omega-3 fatty acids and the brain: "A review of the independent and shared effects of EPA, DPA and DHA". DHA has been shown to promote the differentiation of neural stem cells into neurons and is DHA is quantitatively the most important Omega-3 PUFA in the brain but EPA is playing an equally important part. EPA therapy in Parkinsons models reduced movement restrictions, improved procedural memory issues, and decreased the production of inflammation-inducing cytokines in the striatum. It was observed that EPA not only enhanced cell health but also prevented the formation of cytoplasmic clumps. Additionally, EPA's comprehensive protective qualities include moderating the rise of Tyrosine-related kinase B (TrkB) receptors and reducing the levels of reactive oxygen species and nitric oxide. This protective mechanism may be due to the suppression of neuronal NADPH oxidase and COX-2 by EPA. These findings correlate with abnormal lipid raft signaling and cognitive decline observed during the development of these neurodegenerative disorders. [89, 90]

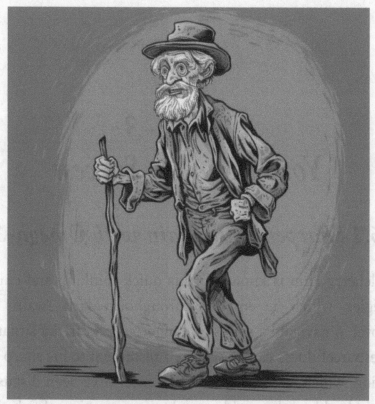

Fig. 30: Can your brain thrive into old age with a 90% Omega-3 deficiency?
Research suggests the seeds of dementia are sown much earlier in life.

Chapter 6

Omega-3
Your Road to Success

6.1 Sharpen Your Brain with Omega-3

Huckleberry Finn is known for his quick thinking and cunning strategies, which he employs throughout Mark Twain's classic novel to navigate a series of dangerous and tricky situations. His resourcefulness can be seen as a testament to his sharp brain function, which, according to the science we've been discussing, could indeed be enhanced by regular consumption of fish rich in Omega-3 fatty acids.

Let's say, in this scenario, Huck has been eating a steady diet of fish, thereby providing his brain with ample Omega-3 fatty acids which are crucial for optimal cognitive function. As his abusive father, Pap, comes searching for him, Huck doesn't just blindly sprint into the forest, putting distance between him and his father but leaving himself lost and vulnerable. Instead, Huck leverages his now Omega-3 boosted brainpower.

He takes a moment to think and comes up with an ingenious plan: he decides to use a pig. By killing the pig and spreading its blood in a deceptive trail, he not only creates a misleading sign of his alleged death but also secures himself a source of food for the upcoming days. This move could be considered a strategic feat that required problem-solving skills, forward-thinking, and quick decision-making—all cognitive functions that can be enhanced by a diet rich in Omega-3 fatty acids.

Now, of course, it's important to note that Omega-3 fatty acids are not the only factor contributing to Huck's wits and resourcefulness. Many other factors, like his natural intelligence, experiences, and inherent resilience, also play crucial roles. But a diet rich in Omega-3 could have potentially given his brain that extra edge needed to navigate the intense challenges of his life.

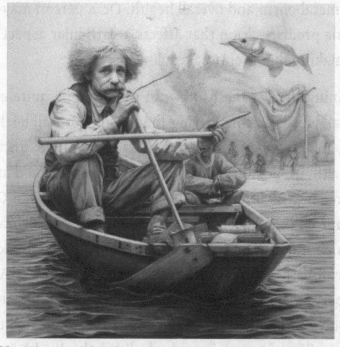

Fig. 31: Hucks' natural fish diet may have helped him to make smarter decisions on his advantageous journey! What is the weakest link in your diet?

The human body is a complex and finely balanced system, and Omega-3 fatty acids are just one piece of a larger nutritional and physiological puzzle. The body needs a variety of nutrients to function properly, and each of these nutrients plays its own vital role.

However, Omega-3 fatty acids are particularly important because they are integral to brain health and function. They contribute to the fluidity of cell membranes, influence signal transduction, and are involved in the regulation of gene expression. If we don't get enough Omega-3, it can impact these processes, leading to potential health problems.

But the weakest link can be different for different individuals and at different times. For example, someone who has a poor diet lacking in several important nutrients could have multiple "weak links" in their metabolism and overall health. Or, a person may have an epigenetic predisposition that affects a particular aspect of their health, making that their weakest link.

Determining the "weakest link" can therefore be quite complex, and usually involves considering the person's overall health, diet, lifestyle, and epigenetics. In the context of cognitive function and brain health, if a person is deficient in Omega-3, it could indeed be considered a weak link. Ensuring an adequate intake of Omega-3 could improve this aspect of health and support overall brain function, which might manifest as better problem-solving skills, like those demonstrated by Huck in your earlier example. As a side note, Albert Einstein was certainly a brilliant mind. But later in life he was advised by his doctors to cut out meat and fish from his diet. Albert Einstein experienced a decline in his health in his later years. In the early 1950s, he began to suffer from various health issues. He had recurring digestive problems, including abdominal pain and digestive disorders, which led to a few surgeries and died of heart disease and an aortic aneurysm.

What is natural intelligence?

When we discuss "natural intelligence," we're usually referring to the inherent capacity of an individual's brain to learn, adapt, problem-solve, and comprehend complex ideas. This includes cognitive abilities such as memory, attention, language, and decision-making. This inherent capacity is determined by a variety of factors, including epigenetics, but also the environment in which one grows and develops.

However, it's important to clarify that having a certain level of natural intelligence doesn't determine an individual's full potential. The brain is an incredibly adaptable organ capable of learning and growing throughout life, a property known as neuroplasticity. This means that through various interventions such as education, brain training exercises, maintaining a healthy lifestyle, and even proper nutrition (like a diet rich in Omega-3 fatty acids), one can significantly improve cognitive functions and overall brain performance.

So, while people might be born with different levels of "natural intelligence," the capacity for growth and improvement is present in everyone. However, how much each person can improve or how they can best optimize their potential can vary greatly, as it depends on a complex interplay of many factors, including epigenetic predispositions, personal circumstances, dedication to learning, and the availability of resources and opportunities.

We can sum up the topic of intelligence with a question: Does everyone with the same access to maximum proper nutrition in the womb and early life plus a loving challenging caretaker have a similar chance at IQ and EQ in life? The development of intelligence (both IQ and EQ) is a complex interplay of both epigenetic and environmental factors, and it's a subject of ongoing debate in the field of psychology and neuroscience.

Epigenetics do play a role in the development of intelligence. Certain epigenetic traits that influence brain development and function can be passed from parents to their children. Therefore, individuals may have certain epigenetic predispositions that impact their cognitive abilities.

However, environmental factors like nutrition, upbringing, and education also play a significant role. Early life experiences and exposure to a stimulating and supportive environment can greatly enhance a child's cognitive development. Proper nutrition, particularly in the womb and during early childhood, is crucial for brain development. Deficiencies in certain nutrients during these critical periods can impair cognitive development, while a balanced, nutrient-rich diet can support it.

Furthermore, emotional intelligence (EQ) is strongly influenced by social and emotional experiences in childhood. Children who grow up in a loving, supportive, and communicative environment are more likely to develop strong emotional intelligence.

However, even with the same access to nutrition and a nurturing environment, there can still be variability in IQ and EQ outcomes due to individual differences in epigenetics, resilience, and personal experiences.

While providing a good start with adequate nutrition and a nurturing environment can certainly enhance the potential for higher IQ and EQ, it doesn't guarantee equal outcomes. There is also the factor of individual effort and the continuous learning and adaptation that humans go through throughout their lives which plays a significant role in the development of these qualities.

Studies have suggested that Omega-3 fatty acids play a crucial role in brain development during fetal and early childhood stages. DHA (Docosahexaenoic Acid), a type of Omega-3 fatty acid, is particularly important for the development of the brain and eyes. [92, 93]

Omega-3 fatty acids, including DHA, are essential for neurodevelopment from the earliest stages of fetal development through to the end of the breastfeeding period. DHA is a primary structural component of the human brain and cerebral cortex. DHA is strongly concentrated in the gray matter of the brain, which is involved in various higher brain functions, such as cognition and memory.

Several studies have found associations between higher maternal intake of fish (which is high in DHA) or Omega-3 supplements during pregnancy and better brain development in their children, as measured by tests of intelligence, language, and motor skills in early childhood. Of course more research is always needed in this area to fully understand the extent and mechanisms of these benefits. But it is clearly the effect of neuronal lipid rafts that influence the healthy communication of the brain neurons in different areas and their inflammatory status.

In conclusion, while Omega-3 fatty acids, such as DHA, are crucial for brain development, they are not the only factor determining a child's future intelligence. Other factors, including epigenetic influences, other nutritional factors, and the overall nurturing environment, also play a substantial role in a child's cognitive development.

An intelligent brain requires high amounts of Omega-3!

The brain is indeed rich in fats, known as lipids. Approximately 60% of the dry weight of the mammalian brain is fat, making it one of the fattiest organs in the body. [79, 136]

Omega-3 fatty acids, particularly docosahexaenoic acid (DHA), represent a significant proportion of these brain lipids. While it's challenging to define the exact percentage of Omega-3 fats in the brain, estimates often cite about 20% of the brain's total fat content is composed of DHA.

DHA is crucial for brain health throughout all stages of life, from supporting neurodevelopment in infants to maintaining cognitive function and preventing neurodegenerative diseases in adults. DHA is highly concentrated in the cell membranes of neurons, where it provides fluidity and influences various cellular processes essential for optimal brain function.

Despite the high natural concentration of DHA in the brain, the body is not efficient at producing DHA on its own. Therefore, it's important to obtain this essential nutrient through dietary sources, such as fatty fish, or through supplementation.

Within this context, it's crucial to highlight the significance of Omega-3 intake during pregnancy and fetal growth, as well as during the baby's first year. Unfortunately blood tests show how the high demand for DHA leaves both the mother and baby highly deficient.

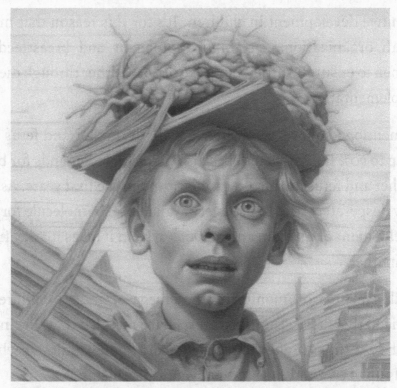
Fig. 32: Being focused and erudite requires brain capacity.

Especially during pregnancy, there's indeed a considerable demand for Omega-3 fatty acids, specifically DHA, because they play a vital role in the development of the baby's brain and nervous system. The fetus is dependent on the mother for its supply of DHA, and this demand can deplete the mother's own stores, potentially leaving both mother and baby deficient if dietary intake isn't sufficient.

One of the primary ways DHA is delivered to the fetus is through the placenta during pregnancy. After birth, infants continue to receive DHA through breast milk. However, if a mother's dietary intake of DHA is low, her ability to pass on sufficient amounts of these important fats can be compromised.

Several studies have shown correlations between the mother's intake of Omega-3 fats during pregnancy and several aspects of cognitive development in children. It's for this reason that many health organizations recommend pregnant and breastfeeding women to ensure a sufficient intake of DHA either through diet or supplementation.

As mentioned above, tests show how both mother and fetus can be up to 90% DHA deficient because of the high demands for both mother and fetus during pregnancies and in the first years. As the baby desperately tries to use every available DHA molecule for the development of its brain and nervous system it takes it away from the mother.

For this very reason, monitoring the Omega-6/3 index in children is particularly crucial. Numerous tests have revealed that this index can be 2-3 times higher in teenagers and young adults, reaching levels up to 60:1 and even 100:1 in youthful athletes.

The reason behind this growing trend of elevated inflammatory indexes in younger generations is uncertain. Still, possible contributors could include increased screen time, which escalates the demand for DHA in the eyes, and epigenetic factors.

What's clear from studies is that during development, a fetus will extract every accessible DHA molecule from the mother and its own EPA reserves to facilitate the growth of its brain and nervous system. For instance, a mother previously identified with a low index was found to be 65% deficient in DHA in the third trimester and shortly after birth, implying that the mother redirects all available DHA to the developing fetus.

Omega-3 fatty acids, particularly DHA (docosahexaenoic acid), have been widely recognized for their critical role in brain health throughout all stages of life, from fetal development and infancy to adulthood and old age.

In early life, adequate Omega-3 intake, particularly DHA, contributes to brain development. Some studies suggest a correlation between Omega-3 intake in pregnant mothers or in early childhood and improved cognitive outcomes, such as higher IQ scores and better reading and memory skills. [93, 135]

During adulthood, Omega-3 fatty acids play a role in maintaining brain function. Regular intake of Omega-3 fatty acids has been linked to reduced risk of depression and improved mental clarity and focus.

As already discussed, in older adults, a consistent intake of Omega-3 fatty acids may be beneficial for maintaining cognitive health and preventing neurodegenerative diseases. Epidemiological studies suggest that people who consume more fish, which is high in Omega-3 fatty acids, have a lower risk of developing Alzheimer's disease and dementia. [137]

It's important to note that while Omega-3 fatty acids are beneficial for brain health, they are not the sole determinant of cognitive function or IQ. Cognitive development and function are multifaceted and can be influenced by numerous other factors, including epigenetics, other nutritional factors, environmental influences, physical activity, and overall health.

In summary, IQ development requires DHA galore! The availability of DHA, one of the major Omega-3 fatty acids, is crucial for the development of the brain and nervous system during fetal development and throughout childhood. DHA plays an integral role in forming neural tissue, particularly in the retina and the brain.

Several research studies have indicated that a sufficient supply of DHA in utero and during early childhood can have significant impacts on cognitive development and intelligence. For instance, a number of studies have shown associations between higher maternal intake of DHA during pregnancy and improved cognitive outcomes in their children. Similarly, supplementation with DHA during infancy and early childhood has also been associated with improved cognitive performance. Basak 2021: "During the last trimester of gestation and for the first 18 months after birth, both (DHA) and arachidonic acid (ARA) are preferentially deposited within the cerebral cortex at a rapid rate. [94]

Conversely, DHA deficiency during these critical periods of development can lead to cognitive deficits and has been associated with conditions like ADHD, dyslexia, and aggressive hostility.

It is also suggested that DHA may have neuroprotective effects and could potentially delay the onset or slow down the progression of cognitive decline in the elderly, including Alzheimer's disease and dementia, although more research is needed in this area.

However, it's important to note that while DHA is a crucial component of brain health and cognitive development, it's not the only factor. epigenetics, overall nutrition, environmental factors, and access to education and stimulation also play significant roles in determining a person's IQ and cognitive health throughout their lifespan.

6.2 How Omega-3 Helps You Work Smarter, Not Harder

Everyone has unproductive days. Nothing seems to be very fruitful no matter what you do on that day—the rhythm of your cognitive attention alternates between periods of focused engagement and moments of mental drifting. Mental attention is a brain function that demands a high degree of effective neural connectivity. The inability to focus is linked to brain inflammation and can be seen as a form of ADHD in the wider sense. We already discussed how Omega-3 affects ADHD and mood disorders in the young. Unfortunately, recent testing shows their brains are 2-3 times more inflammatory than older generations.

Indeed, Omega-3 fatty acids, particularly DHA, play a critical role in the structure and function of brain cells, and they promote healthy brain development and function throughout all stages of life. Insufficient levels of Omega-3 have been linked to various cognitive disorders and mental health conditions, including attention deficit hyperactivity disorder (ADHD), depression, schizophrenia, and dementia.

Omega-3 fatty acids could potentially enhance cognitive function in several ways:

Neurotransmitter function: Omega-3 are involved in the synthesis and function of neurotransmitters, the chemicals that neurons use to communicate with each other. Omega-3 may particularly enhance dopamine and serotonin transmission, which are key neurotransmitters involved in attention, motivation, and mood regulation.

Brain cell structure and flexibility: DHA, a major form of Omega-3 in the brain, is incorporated into the cell membranes of neurons, enhancing their fluidity. This allows for better communication between neurons, which may improve cognitive functions such as memory, focus, and decision-making.

Anti-inflammatory effects: Omega-3 have powerful anti-inflammatory properties, which can protect the brain from damage and aging by reducing neuroinflammation. Chronic inflammation is thought to be a major contributor to cognitive decline, mood disorders, and neurodegenerative diseases.

Brain-derived neurotrophic factor (BDNF): Omega-3 can increase the production of BDNF [138], a protein that promotes the survival of nerve cells by playing a role in growth, differentiation, and maintenance of neurons in the central nervous system. Higher BDNF levels are associated with better memory and mood.

In conclusion, ensuring adequate intake of Omega-3, whether through diet or supplementation, could potentially improve cognitive performance, focus, mood, and overall brain health.

Tests show that younger generations are testing at inflammatory indices Omega-6/3 over 40:1 and even worse if they are athletes. The demands for DHA in the youth due to increased screen time and simultaneous lack of nutrition and increased consumption of processed foods probably lies at the basis of this testing debacle.

6.3 Inspiring Success Stories: Omega-3, *the stress reducer*

Biomarkers of stress response in humans can be classified into several categories based on the physiological systems they are associated with. Here are some examples of stress markers influenced by Omega-3 that can all be measured by blood tests. In other words, in addition to the Omega-6/3 index test you should see these markers reduced with proper Omega-3 supplementation:

Cortisol: Often referred to as the "stress hormone," it is released by the adrenal glands in response to stress. Cortisol levels are often measured in blood, saliva, or urine.

Adrenocorticotropic Hormone (ACTH): Released by the pituitary gland to stimulate the production of cortisol by the adrenal glands.

Autonomic Nervous System Biomarkers: These are substances related to the automatic responses of the body to stress, including heart rate variability and blood pressure.

Epinephrine (Adrenaline) and Norepinephrine (Noradrenaline): These hormones are released during acute stress to prepare the body for "fight or flight."

Immune System Biomarkers: Chronic stress can affect the immune system and this is reflected in the levels of certain immune-related substances.

C-Reactive Protein (CRP): An elevated level of CRP is seen in response to inflammation in the body.

Interleukins (IL-6, IL-10), Tumor Necrosis Factor-alpha (TNF-alpha): These are cytokines, substances released by immune cells in response to stress or inflammation.

Metabolic Biomarkers: Chronic stress can cause changes in metabolism that can be measured through certain markers.

Neuroendocrine Biomarkers: These are substances released in response to stress by the brain and the endocrine system.

Glucose: Chronic stress can lead to elevated glucose levels.

Lipids: Stress can cause changes in lipid metabolism, including increased levels of triglycerides and LDL cholesterol.

Psychological/Behavioral Biomarkers: While these aren't substances that can be measured in a lab, behaviors and psychological states associated with stress can be tracked as biomarkers.

Mood and Anxiety: Questionnaires can be used to assess mood and anxiety levels.

Cognitive Function: Stress can impact cognitive abilities like memory and attention, which can be measured using cognitive tests.

Researchers agree: "Reducing cortisol levels are among the most important goals for general health".

Omega-3 lowers cortisol levels! But only at higher dosages! Cortisol, a hormone released by the adrenal gland in response to stress and helps to regulate blood sugar levels, blood pressure, and the immune system throughout the entire day.

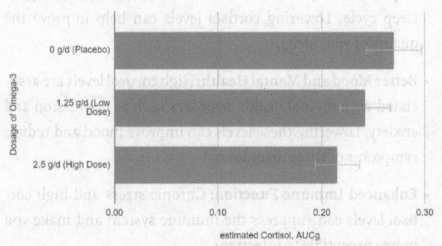

Fig. 33: Adapted from Madison (2021): "Omega-3 supplementation reduced total cortisol levels throughout the stressor. The high dose of Omega-3 (2.5 g/d), but not the low dose (1.25 g/d), produced a significant (19%) reduction in total cortisol release compared to the placebo group. [95]

To avoid systemic inflammation and the resulting metabolic diseases including hypertension, diabetes, cardiovascular disease and even cancer it is imperative to keep average cortisol level low.

Stress biomarkers can be measured by blood tests

Cortisol, also known as the "stress hormone," plays a crucial role in various functions, including metabolism, immune response, and the body's response to stress. It's necessary for survival and helps your body respond to danger. However, persistently high levels of cortisol — often as a result of chronic stress — can lead to numerous health problems.

Reducing chronic high cortisol levels can have several benefits for your health, such as:

- **Improved Sleep:** High cortisol levels can interfere with your sleep cycle. Lowering cortisol levels can help improve the quality of your sleep.

- **Better Mood and Mental Health:** High cortisol levels are associated with mental health disorders such as depression and anxiety. Lowering these levels can improve mood and reduce symptoms of these disorders.

- **Enhanced Immune Function:** Chronic stress and high cortisol levels can suppress the immune system and make you more susceptible to infections.

- **Improved Metabolic Health:** High cortisol levels can lead to weight gain and increased risk of metabolic syndrome, a cluster of conditions that increase the risk of heart disease, stroke, and type 2 diabetes.

Reducing cortisol levels is crucial for maintaining overall health and wellbeing. Cortisol, often referred to as the "stress hormone," is produced by the adrenal glands in response to stress and low blood-glucose concentration. While it's essential for helping the body respond to stress, prolonged high levels can lead to various health problems, including anxiety, depression, heart disease, weight gain, and trouble sleeping. There are several ways to reduce cortisol levels and improve your health. These include regular physical activity, maintaining a healthy diet, ensuring adequate sleep, practicing mindfulness and relaxation techniques like yoga and meditation, and fostering strong social connections. By managing stress and keeping cortisol levels in check, you can promote better physical and mental health.

To reduce cortisol levels, also consider the following:

- **Regular Exercise:** Regular physical activity can reduce cortisol levels and improve your mood. Especially outdoor activities are important connect your body with Nature.

- **Balanced Diet:** Consuming a balanced Protein/Fat/Carbohydrate diet with sufficient amounts of all essential nutrients can help your body better cope with stress. Intermittent fasting but regular meals are crucial. Avoid processed foods high in Omega-6 at all costs.

- **Stress Management Techniques:** Practices like Qi Gong, yoga, meditation, mindfulness, and deep breathing can help reduce stress and lower cortisol levels.

- **Adequate Sleep:** Prioritize getting enough quality sleep each night. Lack of sleep can raise cortisol levels. See a sleep specialist if you are battling insomnia.

- **Social Connections:** Spending quality time with friends and family, connecting with others, and having fun can also help lower cortisol levels. Be present.

Chapter 7

How to Get More Omega-3?

7.1 Finding Omega-3: Where to Look and What to Eat and Easy Ways to Add Omega-3 to Your Everyday Meals

How do you go about getting a good Omega-3 supply incorporated into your diet? Do you know where your Omega-3 comes from and if it is rancid? What are the absolute amounts of Omega-6 in those foods?

Traditionally, the only safe foods humans consumed are fresh fish and grass-fed-grass-finished beef as the major source for Omega-3 since the Neolithic Agricultural Revolution. Of course eating wild game is ideal but returning to a hunter/gatherer life-style seems impossible at this point although the availability of wild-game or venison is certainly an option at times.

Here are some strategies to ensure you're getting a quality Omega-3 supply in your diet:

- **Eat Fatty Fish:** Consuming fatty fish like salmon, mackerel, sardines, and trout at least twice a week can provide a good amount of both EPA and DHA, two types of Omega-3 that are crucial for heart, brain, and eye health.

- **Grass-fed Meat:** Grass-fed beef is a good source of Omega-3 if it is grass finished, much better than grain-fed alternatives. This also applies to other types of grass-fed meat like lamb and venison.

- **Chia and Flax Seeds:** These seeds are excellent sources of ALA, another type of Omega-3. However, keep in mind that ALA needs to be converted into EPA and DHA in your body to be effective, and this conversion process can be inefficient.

- **Omega-3 Fortified Foods:** Some foods are fortified with Omega-3, such as eggs and yogurt. However it is unlikely that such procedures ensure the Omega-3 is not turned rancid in such processed foods. Remember it is a very fragile molecule and oxidizes quickly if not stabilized within whole foods. For that same reason it is unlikely that your pets receive any significant amount of stable Omega-3 in the commercially available pet foods.

- **Seaweed and Algae:** If you're a vegetarian or vegan, these can be excellent sources of Omega-3. You can find them in various forms such as supplements, snacks, or as ingredients for vegan sushi.

- **Walnuts:** These nuts are a good plant-based source of Omega-3. However they only contain a significant amount of ALA and little or no EPA or DHA. In addition processed, peeled and packaged nuts probably only contain Omega-6.

- **Supplements:** You most likely will find it difficult to incorporate enough Omega-3 through your diet and you need to consider high-quality stabilized supplements.

Do your research and choose a reputable brand to ensure you're getting a quality non-rancid product. Probably the only way to find out if your supplement is working properly may be a regular blood-RBC fatty acid test (eg. after 6 months). However, experimenting with inferior products causes you to lose valuable time. Tests show that unfortunately most products are rancid (see appendix). To my current knowledge as of 2023, only Zinzino, Eqology and Norsan show significant test improvements. Other reputable Omega-3 brands may be available, however it is not always easy to verify what criteria 3rd party food-lab tests actually use to evaluate products.

Here are some additional suggestions on choosing supplements: #1 the product needs to contain significant amounts of antioxidants (Vitamin E and D alone are not sufficient); #2 the product needs to have a verified low TOTOX value (discussed below) and #3 gel capsules are usually inferior to larger liquid bottles due to the increased risk of oxygen exposure.

If you are a vegetarian or vegan, the only way you will be able to to get EPA or DHA is by your own enzymatic conversion of ALA (Alpha-linolenic acid) which you can get for eg. non-rancid flax seeds. There are efforts to produce vegan sourced Omega-3 from algae however these oils currently have similar or worse rancidity and storage problems and also a much lower amount of EPA. In addition, these algae-produced oils lack rare Omega-3 species that are only present in reasonable amounts in fresh cold water fish.

Look for more tables of Omega-3 content in various foods in the appendix. But certainly on the top of the list are properly preserved sardines, mackerel or salmon. Fish roe is also an option as well. The warmer climate the fish lives in and larger it is, the less its Omega-3 content. Shellfish should be reduced to a minimum due to its allergenic properties.

Beef should be grass-fed-grass-finished (not on a feedlot). Beef should be fresh or flash frozen at very cold temperatures and only thawed once. When it comes to the quality of poultry or pork: it depends on what the animals were fed. In general, the inflammatory index of these meats is higher due to the grain and seed feeds.

In addition, seeds should be freshly processed or flash frozen. Nuts should be fresh, non-processed and still preserved in their original shell. In general, except for walnuts, all nuts are highly inflammatory. Also pay attention to the absolute amounts of inflammatory Omega-6 and not just the inflammatory index ratio. Examples can be found in the appendix. For example walnuts are considered to be an Omega-3 superfood. However they contain a fair amount of Omega-6 as well (up to 38%). So if the Omega-3 content is rancid, the end result is inflammatory.

All vegetable oils are highly inflammatory! Cook with saturated fats such as lard, butter and coconut. Only use Olive or Avocado oils sparingly as they still have larger amounts of Omega-6.

Please check the appendix for Omega-6 contents of common plants and animal foods.

7.2 The Right Source and Time for Omega-3 Supplements

The Right source for Omega-3 Supplements is the one that shows a benefit of an improved Omega-6/3 index. After 5-9 months you should test your RBC membranes (not liquid blood) for this index and it should be largely improved and below 4:1. Often you can tell the rancidity of your supplement by opening up a gel cap and smell. If you the product causes indigestion and burping it most likely is rancid. Supplements have to be stabilized against oxidation by proper anti-oxidants, Vitamin E and D are not efficient enough for this purpose as their redox potential is too low.

Rancid Omega-3 supplements can contain oxidized lipids. Oxidation is a chemical reaction that happens when oils or fats react with oxygen. It's a natural process that can occur in any oil, including Omega-3 fatty acids, and is accelerated by exposure to heat, light, or oxygen.

Oxidized Omega-3 fatty acids can lead to the formation of harmful compounds, such as:

Peroxides and hydroperoxides: These are the primary oxidation products and are unstable, further breaking down into secondary products.

Aldehydes, ketones, and alkenals: These secondary products are more stable and can accumulate in the oil. They can be harmful even in small amounts. Aldehydes, in particular, have been associated with increased risk of heart disease and other conditions.

Trans fats: While this is more common in industrially processed fats, some oxidation processes can lead to the formation of trans fats, which are associated with heart disease and other health problems.

Consuming rancid oils can cause digestive distress, such as diarrhea or cramps. In the long term, it can lead to increased oxidative stress and inflammation, which are risk factors for many chronic diseases, including heart disease and cancer. [96, 138]

Therefore, it's important to store Omega-3 supplements as recommended by the manufacturer, usually in a cool, dark place, and to consume them before the expiration date. Quality is also crucial; buy your supplements from reputable sources that can provide evidence of third-party testing for oxidation and so called TOTOX values.

TOTOX value (Total Oxidation) is a measurement commonly used to assess the freshness and quality of oils, including Omega-3 supplements. It's a composite measure of primary and secondary oxidation products in the oil. TOTOX is calculated using the following formula: TOTOX = 2 x PV (Peroxide Value) + AV (Anisidine Value)

The Peroxide Value (PV) indicates the level of primary oxidation products, which are the initial by-products produced when fats and oils begin to oxidize. These compounds can degrade into secondary oxidation products.

The Anisidine Value (AV) measures secondary oxidation products, such as aldehydes, that are formed as the primary products further degrade. These compounds are responsible for the rancid smells and tastes associated with spoiled oils and can be harmful if ingested.

In general, a lower TOTOX value indicates a fresher, higher-quality oil. The Global Organization for EPA and DHA Omega-3 (GOED) has set the maximum allowable TOTOX value for Omega-3 oils at 26. Anything above this value is considered not suitable for consumption.

In summary, I would not recommend a product that does not show 3rd party TOTOX value testing results and the improvements of Omega-6/3 index via 3rd party blood testing.

Conclusion: Your Journey to a Happier, Healthier, More Successful Life

Unfortunately, humans have not evolved quickly enough to produce adequate amounts of these fatty acid molecules. In our history on this planet, we have always relied on other species, namely grazing animals and fish, to give us this supply of nutrients.

The role of Omega-3 fatty acids in human health and evolution is incredibly significant. Humans are unable to synthesize these essential fats in our bodies, which means that we must obtain them through our diets. Historically, our ancestors likely received ample Omega-3 from a varied diet rich in wild game, fish, and other seafood, as well as certain plants and seeds.

Today, the typical Western diet is heavily skewed toward Omega-6 fatty acids, found in abundance in processed and fast foods. While Omega-6 fats are essential in moderation, an imbalanced Omega-6 to Omega-3 ratio has been linked to a host of health issues, from heart disease and diabetes to cognitive decline and mood disorders.

It is therefore crucial to be mindful of our intake of these critical nutrients and strive for a balanced Omega-6 to Omega-3 ratio. This can be achieved by consuming a diet rich in Omega-3 sources like fatty fish (salmon, mackerel, sardines), flaxseeds, chia seeds, walnuts, and Omega-3 fortified eggs, or by taking high-quality Omega-3 supplements. Regular testing of Omega-3 levels can help individuals track their progress and adjust their diet or supplement regimen as necessary.

In my opinion and as a large body of research shows, Omega-3 fatty acids is the most vital component of human health and evolution, underscoring the need for proper nutrition and balance in our modern diets.

Both Omega-3 and Vitamin D are now considered the most important *neutraceuticals*. A nutraceutical is a term derived from the combination of the words "Nutrition" and "Pharmaceutical." It refers to a food or food component that provides health benefits beyond basic nutritional value, often with the potential to prevent or treat various diseases and health conditions. Nutraceuticals can be naturally occurring in foods or created through a manufacturing process and added to foods or consumed as supplements.

Omega-3 is 'life' as it keeps the lipid membrane alive and the functionality of all cells rely on it.

Omega-3 has direct effects on: Vision and eye health, Immune Function and Inflammation control, Cell division, Mitochondrial energy production, Liver Detoxification, Reproduction, Brain and Nerve health, Wound Healing and Stem Cell function, Bone-Tendon-Muscle Regeneration, Heart and Lung health, Athletic performance, Digestion, Blood pressure and Kidney Health, Sugar metabolism, Hearing, Memory, Mental Clarity and many more. REDUCTION of INFLAMMATION lies at the center of the mechanism of these chronic diseases! In addition humans living above the 36th latitude are prone to be highly Vitamin D deficient and even in sunny climates people now avoid sunshine because of the fear of cancer.

Modern Nutritionists agree: "Including a variety of Omega-3-rich fish in your diet provides numerous health benefits, such as improved cardiovascular health, reduced inflammation, and better cognitive function."

Please don't just take my word for it! Read peer reviewed clinical studies and test your inflammatory Omega-6/3 index and Vitamin D levels regularly.

Finally, once you have taken the time to restore your brain and heart to near capacity, a process that may take up to a year or longer, it's time to use it. As discussed, some of your organ stem cells take a long time to exchange, so be patient and don't be surprised by the changes that will happen in your general health and the newly found levels of concentration, determination and stamina. Use methods such as the Silva method [100] to further the development of your right brain and enter new realms of functionality in your life that you have not explored. Don't be afraid to push your body to new limits in exercising and the mountains that you always wanted to climb.

And lastly, please remember that Omega-3 fish oil is a nature-given nutraceutical, not an artificial pharmaceutical, although there are efforts developing it into a drug. These artificial Omega-3 molecules continue to show serious side effects. In general, for the same reason you should avoid processed foods, I recommend avoiding chemical drugs at all costs!

Appendix

Bonus A

Your Go-To List of Omega-3 Rich Foods

Why fish oils are the better source for Omega-3?

We already provided Omega-3 content of common foods in chapter 2.1. However, plant foods only contain ALA-Omega-3 and your body would need to convert them to EPA and DHA enzymatically.

Fish obtain their EPA and DHA from algae. Here is how that works. Algae, including microalgae, are significant sources of Omega-3 fatty acids, particularly eicosapentaenoic acid (EPA) and docosahexaenoic acid (DHA). The synthesis of EPA and DHA in algae involves the conversion of simple fatty acids into more complex ones. The process is catalyzed by a series of enzymes, such as desaturases, which introduce double bonds into the fatty acid chain, and elongases, which lengthen the chain.

The synthesis of these fatty acids in algae occurs in the chloroplasts (the site of photosynthesis) and the endoplasmic reticulum (a structure involved in the production of lipids and proteins). It begins with the production of alpha-linolenic acid (ALA), a short-chain Omega-3 fatty acid. This is then converted into stearidonic acid (SDA), then to EPA, and finally to DHA, through the actions of the desaturase and elongase enzymes, similar to the conversion process in humans, however at a much more efficient rate. Photosynthesis provides the energy that algae need to grow and synthesize a variety of compounds, including EPA and DHA. The energy from sunlight is captured and converted into chemical energy, which fuels these biosynthetic processes.

Additionally, the fatty acids produced by algae, including EPA and DHA, are integrated into the chloroplast membrane (and the analog mitochondria). This improves the fluidity and functionality of the membrane, which in turn aids in the photosynthesis process. Thus, the synthesis of these fatty acids is both a result of and a contributor to the process of photosynthesis in algae.

Why is Omega-3 stable in algae?

Phlorotannins are a group of tannins found in brown algae, known for their strong antioxidant properties. These compounds are believed to have the capacity to prevent the oxidation of Omega-3 fatty acids, which enhances the stability and shelf-life of the fish oil. However, as far as the stabilization of Omega-3 within the bodies of living fish, it's crucial to note that the fish do not necessarily stabilize Omega-3 fats using phlorotannins. Their bodies are constantly metabolizing these fats for use in various cellular functions, and their fresh consumption (or immediate processing and appropriate storage in the case of fish oil) mitigates the opportunity for oxidation.

Processing Fish oil requires strong antioxidants. Both phlorotannins and olive polyphenols have demonstrated high antioxidant activity. Vitamin E or D or ascorbate are not sufficient.

Fish	Omega-3 (grams per 100g)	Omega-6 (grams per 100g)	Omega-6/Omega-3 ratio
Salmon	2.6	0.2	0.08
Mackerel	2.7	0.05	0.02
Tuna	1.1	0.09	0.08
Sardines	1.7	0.14	0.08
Trout	1.2	0.4	0.33
Herring	1.7	0.2	0.12
Halibut	0.4	0.1	0.25

Table: Omega-6/3 index compared.

Please note that these numbers are just estimates and they can vary depending on many factors, including the age of the fish, their diet, the water temperature, and the specific species of the fish. Always aim to consume fish from sustainable sources to maintain the health of our oceans.

Fish Species	DHA (mg)	EPA (mg)	Total Omega-3 (mg)
Salmon (Atlantic)	1425	774	2199
Mackerel (Atlantic)	982	698	1680
Herring (Atlantic)	944	710	1654
Sardines (Atlantic)	509	473	982
Trout (Rainbow)	859	277	1136
Tuna (Albacore)	751	228	979
Anchovies	694	211	905
Arctic Char	763	134	897
Halibut	534	134	668
Cod (Pacific)	129	193	322
Tilapia	111	40	151

Table: DHA and EPA amounts of different fish species (approximations).

Nuts are generally inflammatory

Nuts are rich in unsaturated fats which are susceptible to oxidation. Once the nut is peeled or cracked open, these fats are exposed to oxygen, light, and heat, all of which can speed up the process of oxidation, leading to rancidity. Hence, pre-peeled or cracked nuts can potentially go rancid faster than those in shells.

The problem is that nuts contain far more Omega-6 than Omega-3 to begin with and Omega-3 is easiest to oxidize. So, its it best to only use whole nuts and crack them yourself.

The stability of a nut without its shell varies depending on several factors, including the type of nut, how it's stored, and the environmental conditions it's exposed to.

To prolong their shelf-life and avoid rancidity, nuts should be stored in a cool, dark, and dry place. Refrigeration or freezing can further prolong their freshness. Vacuum sealing or packaging in an inert gas can also reduce oxidation.

However, it's important to note that even with these precautions, nuts can still eventually turn rancid due to the natural degradation of the fats they contain.

Also, it's worth noting that rancidity does not mean that the food is unsafe to eat. Rancidity primarily affects taste and smell. However, consuming rancid food may not provide the same nutritional benefits as fresh food, and may contain potentially harmful compounds produced during the oxidation process.

It's also important to note that commercially packed nut mixes may also contain added oils, sweeteners, or salt that can affect the stability and potential rancidity of the product.

If you notice a change in the smell or taste of the nuts (they may smell like paint or have a bitter or sour taste), it is best not to consume them as they are likely rancid.

Here is a table of the 10 most commonly consumed nuts, including almonds and peanuts, showing their approximate alpha-linolenic acid (ALA) and Omega-6 fatty acid content. The values are presented per 100 grams (3.5 ounces) of nuts.

Nut Type	Omega-3 (g/100g)	Omega-6 (g/100g)	Omega-6/3 Ratio
Walnuts	9.08	38.09	4.2
Almonds	0.0035	12.07	3448
Pistachios	0.173	13.455	77.8
Cashews	0.062	7.782	125.5
Hazelnuts	0.025	7.92	316.8
Brazil nuts	0.018	20.577	1143.2
Pine nuts	0.095	33.8	355.8
Pecans	1.0	21.6	21.6
Macadamias	0.058	1.5	25.9
Peanuts	0.0034	15.56	4576

Table: The inflammatory Omega-6/3 index increases as the fragile Omega-3 oxidizes and Omega-6 becomes relatively enriched.

Table of common Vegetable oils.

Approximate breakdown of the composition of vegetable oils (amounts are per 100g of oil):

Oil Type	Omega-3 (g)	Omega-6 (g)	Omega-9 (g)	Saturated Fat (g)
Coconut	0	1.8	6	87
Palm	0.2	9.7	42.8	49.3
Olive	0.8	9.8	73	14
Avocado	1	9.8	67	20
Peanut	0	32	47	17
Canola	9.1	28.1	56.1	7.4
Rice Bran	1.2	35	38.4	25
Corn	1.2	52.9	27.6	15
Cottonseed	0	51.5	18.5	26
Grape Seed	0.1	69.6	16.1	10
Sunflower	0.2	65.7	19.5	10
Soy	7.0	50.4	22.8	15.6

Table: These amounts are approximations and the exact values can vary based on the extraction method, refinement process, and other factors.

How the Omega-6/3 test works

Very important: an Omega-3 blood test should always be done on testing the long term RBC (red blood cell) membranes. A "liquid blood" test is not representative of your health status. It can fluctuate greatly depending on recent diet.

The Omega-3 fatty acid levels in blood can be assessed using a dried blood spot (DBS) test. The test is straightforward and non-invasive, making it particularly suitable for clinic and "at home".

Oil Type	Omega-6/3 Ratio	Saturated Fat (%)
Coconut	(No Omega-3)	87
Palm	48.5	49.3
Olive	12.25	14
Avocado	9.8	20
Peanut	(No Omega-3)	17
Canola	3.09	7.4
Rice Bran	29.2	25
Corn	44.1	15
Cottonseed	N/A	26
Grape Seed	696	10
Sunflower	328.5	10
Soy	7.2	15.6

Table: Table comparison of inflammatory Omega-6/3 index compared to saturated fat amount.

Here's how it typically works:

A small prick is made on your finger with a lancet, similar to a glucose test for diabetics. However unlike these glucose tests not the liquid blood but the RBC membranes are tested in the lab.

- A drop of blood is then placed onto a specially prepared card.

- The card is left to dry for several minutes.

- Once dried, the card can be mailed back to a lab in a special envelope, without the need for refrigeration.

- At the lab, the dried blood spots are analyzed for Omega-3 fatty acids, including EPA and DHA. The levels are usually reported as a percentage of total fatty acids.

The Omega-3 index, or the combined percentage of EPA and DHA, is commonly used to assess the Omega-3 status in the blood. A higher Omega-3 index is generally associated with a lower risk of heart diseases.

This kind of testing is useful because it can be done at home and the sample remains stable during transport to the lab. However, it's important to note that like all tests, it is subject to some degree of variability, and results should be interpreted in the context of an individual's overall health and lifestyle.

The Omega-3 index, or the combined percentages of EPA and DHA, are commonly used to assess the Omega-3 status in the blood. A higher Omega-3 index is generally associated with a lower risk of heart diseases but the results are not linear; the thresholds are set at +8%, this typically equates to an index of Omega-6/3 of lower than 4:1.

The average natural level of EPA in the blood is recommended at 3.6%, while that of DHA is 4.7%, and combined they need to be above 8%, preferably 10%. The daily requirement of marine Omega-3 EPA and DHA depends on body type and demand. Eg. an athlete has a much higher demand on DHA. Over 90% of the population tests with indices of much below 4%. Adults weighing 80 kg need to consume approximately 3 grams of Omega-3 (EPA + DHA) daily to get their Omega-3 (EPA + DHA) level above 8%.

Bonus B

Frequently asked Questions About Omega-3 Supplements

For detailed Omega-3 science visit: Omega3health.us/science/

Additional Reads and Resources for which supplements work and which dont and a nutritional guide on Your Omega-3 Journey

What can you do to improve your life in simple easy steps without the stress of having to remember 50 supplements every day and to eat regular good foods? Here are some strategies to remember to take your supplements daily:

Link with a Habit: Pair taking your supplements with a habit that's already firmly established in your daily routine. It could be brushing your teeth, having breakfast, or even after your shower.

Set Reminders: Use technology to your advantage. Set a daily reminder or alarm on your phone or smart device. There are also many apps available specifically designed to help people remember to take their medications and supplements.

Visible Location: Keep your supplements in a place where you'll see them every day, like on your bedside table, kitchen counter, or near your coffee maker.

If you absolutely can't keep track of too many pills you can Use a Pill Organizer: These are handy tools, especially if you have multiple supplements to take. They not only help you remember to take them, but also help you track whether you've already taken them each day.

Incorporate into Meals: If your supplements need to be taken with food, make it a routine to take them during one of your regular meals.

Leverage Routine: If you have a fairly consistent daily routine, try to fit your supplements into this existing structure. For example, if you always have a shot-glass visible at your dinner table. Take your liquid Omega-3 oil with a 50/50 water mixture.

Note: we recommend always taking supplements with food and not on an empty stomach.

Remember, it takes time to form a new habit. Stick with it and soon it will become a normal part of your daily routine.

For more supplements science, visit Omega3health.us/do-supplements-work. For a comprehensive search on general food supplement and nutritional facts you can look here: www.webmd.com/diet/health-benefits-flaxseed

Bonus C

Fat Science: Lipids and Cholesterol

Lets have a look at what lipids really do in the body. According to a study published in the Journal of Lipid Research, lipids constitute about 40% of the dry weight of a typical mammalian cell! Lipids are a group of naturally occurring molecules that include fats, waxes, sterols, monoglycerides, diglycerides, triglycerides. Even fat-soluble vitamins (such as vitamins A, D, E, and K) can be considered lipids. But in general, membrane lipids such as phospholipids each with different lengths and degrees of saturation, as well as numerous glycerolipids and glycerophospholipids are all created by combining different fatty acids with a glycerol backbone.

There are over 1000 species of lipids: Eg. Sphingolipids, which are found primarily in the cell membranes of the nervous system, and sterol lipids, like cholesterol, add even more diversity to the lipid family. They all are important for the many different biological functions including storing energy, insulating the body, and forming cell membranes.

Lipids are characterized by their inability to dissolve in water (they are hydrophobic). Instead, they function as soap like molecules and can only be dissolved in organic solvents like chloroform and some alcohols.

The main biological functions of lipids include:

- Energy Storage: Lipids, particularly triglycerides, are a highly concentrated form of energy storage. When the body needs energy and it is not immediately available from glucose in the bloodstream, it will use lipids to meet energy needs.

- Cell Membrane Structure: Lipids, specifically phospholipids, make up the primary structure of cell membranes. They form a lipid bilayer, with the polar (hydrophilic) heads of the phospholipids facing outward towards the water-based environment, and the nonpolar (hydrophobic) tails facing inward. This structure creates a semi-permeable membrane that allows for the regulation of substances entering and exiting the cell.

- Insulation and Protection: Fat in the body serves to insulate and protect organs, as well as insulate the body to maintain body temperature.

- Hormone Production: Some types of lipids, such as cholesterol, play an essential role in the production of hormones, including steroid hormones like estrogen and testosterone.

- Vitamin Absorption: Dietary fats help in the absorption of the fat-soluble vitamins A, D, E, and K in the intestines. These vitamins are crucial for a variety of bodily functions, including bone health, vision, and blood clotting.

In the cellular membrane a lipid plays an important role with several key functions

- Structural Integrity: Lipids form the main structural component of cell membranes, with phospholipids being the most abundant. These have a hydrophilic (water-attracting) head and two hydrophobic (water-repelling) tails. The result is a phospholipid bilayer, where the hydrophilic heads face outwards and the hydrophobic tails face each other. This structure forms a barrier between the cell and its external environment, while allowing for flexibility and fluidity of the cell membrane.

- Regulation of Membrane Permeability: The lipid bilayer determines what substances can pass into and out of a cell. Small, non-polar molecules can often pass directly through the lipid bilayer, while ions and larger, polar molecules require specific transport proteins.

- Signal Transduction: Lipids can also be involved in signal transduction across the membrane. Certain lipids can act as signaling molecules themselves or as part of a larger signaling complex. For example, phospholipids can be cleaved to form secondary messengers in response to extracellular signals.

- Membrane Protein Function: Lipids in the cell membrane can influence the function of membrane proteins by affecting their structure, localization, and interactions with other molecules.

- Energy Storage as already mentioned: Certain types of lipids, such as triglycerides, are important for energy storage.

- Role of Cholesterol: In animal cells, cholesterol is a crucial component of the cell membrane. It regulates the fluidity of the membrane and prevents fatty acid chains from sticking together, thereby preventing the membrane from becoming too rigid or too fluid.

- Formation of Lipid Rafts: Certain lipids can cluster together with specific proteins to form lipid rafts, which are involved in various cellular processes such as signal transduction, protein sorting, and membrane trafficking.

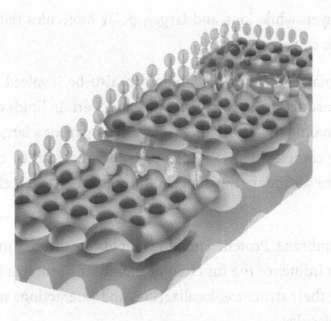

Fig. 34: Lipid rafts are floating in a cell membrane bilayer. Think about the cell membrane as a layer of fluid lipid fats; it is passively held together in weak hydrophobic interactions and rafts of protein-lipid complexes are floating around. These lipid rafts require a good supply of Omega-3.

Examples of lipid species

- Phosphatidylethanolamines (PE): These are a class of phospholipids found in biological membranes. They are synthesized by all living cells and are particularly prominent in nervous tissues. PE aids in membrane fusion and in disassembly of the contractile ring during cytokinesis. Rich in DHA, an important Omega-3 fatty acid that supports brain health.

- Phosphatidylcholines (PC): These are a class of phospholipids that incorporate choline as a headgroup. They are a major component of biological membranes and can also be used in the production of liposomes and lipid bilayers. PC is often found in the outer leaflet of the cell membrane.

- Phosphatidylserine (PS): This is a phospholipid component of the cell membrane. It plays a key role in cell cycle signaling, specifically in relation to apoptosis (programmed cell death). When a cell undergoes apoptosis, PS is no longer restricted to the intracellular side of the membrane and flips to the extracellular surface of the cell, signaling macrophages to engulf the cells.

- Phosphatidylinositol (PI): This class of phospholipid is present in all animal and plant cells. PI forms the basis of a number of important cellular processes, specifically signal transduction pathways. The phosphorylated forms of PI, known as phosphoinositides, play crucial roles in lipid signaling, cell signaling, and membrane trafficking.

Specifically, Phospholipids are a class of lipids that are a major component of all cell membranes. They can form lipid bilayers because of their amphiphilic characteristic and each "head" has a different function to direct the cell in the body, interact with neighboring proteins and signal hormonal messages. Each cell organelle and each different functional cell requires the proper nutrients to form its head group and the proper Omega-3. When Omega-3 is not available the lipid is 'downgraded' to Omega-6, Omega-9 or cholesterol. Research shows the cells most always prefer Omega-3 over Omega-6 and only a certain portion can be saturated fat to keep the membrane fluid and rafts functional. Omega-3 and Omega-6 fatty acids are types of polyunsaturated fats (PUFAs). PUFAs are crucial for creating flexible and fluid cell membranes, which allows for proper cellular functioning including division, communication, and transportation of materials in and out of the cell. They also help create lipid rafts, which are microdomains in the cell membrane that facilitate cellular signaling.

The human body can't produce Omega-3 and Omega-6 fatty acids, which is why they're referred to as essential fatty acids. They need to be obtained from our diet. While both types of fatty acids are important for health, maintaining a proper balance between Omega-6 and Omega-3 is crucial. An imbalance, specifically a diet high in Omega-6 and low in Omega-3, can contribute to systemic inflammation and chronic diseases.

Saturated fats, on the other hand, can cause cell membranes to become more rigid if they are present in high amounts. This can disrupt cellular functions and may contribute to the development of various health problems including heart disease and stroke. Therefore, while saturated fats are not inherently bad and are needed in some amount for optimal membrane health, their intake should be balanced with the intake of unsaturated fats, including Omega-3 and Omega-6 fatty acids.

The formation and functionality of membrane structures like endosomes rely on the fluidity and flexibility provided by poly-unsaturated fatty acids (PUFAs), such as Omega-3 and Omega-6. These fatty acids are often found on the outer layer of the lipid bilayer, providing the necessary flexibility for endocytosis, a process that involves the membrane bending inward to form a pocket, or vesicle, that transports substances into the cell.

On the other hand, the inner layer of the lipid bilayer tends to be more populated with saturated fatty acids. These have straighter chains and pack more tightly together, providing structure and stability to the membrane.

This asymmetric distribution of fatty acids in the lipid bilayer and the balance between saturated and unsaturated fats is critical for the membrane's overall function and health. It impacts not only processes like endocytosis but also various other membrane functions, such as signal transduction, protein function, and the formation of lipid rafts.

During exocytosis, a process where the cell transports molecules out of the cell within vesicles, the lipid bilayer of the vesicle has to merge with the cell's outer membrane. This process requires the formation of a convex structure on the membrane's cytoplasmic side.

To achieve this, the lipid bilayer must have a particular composition that allows it to bend in the appropriate way. In general, the side of the bilayer that favors curvature (in this case, the inner layer during exocytosis) tends to have a greater concentration of saturated fatty acids, which facilitate the formation of the convex shape. The other layer (in this case, the outer layer during exocytosis) will have more polyunsaturated fatty acids, such as Omega-3 and Omega-6, contributing to the overall flexibility of the membrane.

Therefore, a balanced and specific distribution of these different types of fatty acids is crucial for the cell's ability to perform processes like exocytosis effectively.

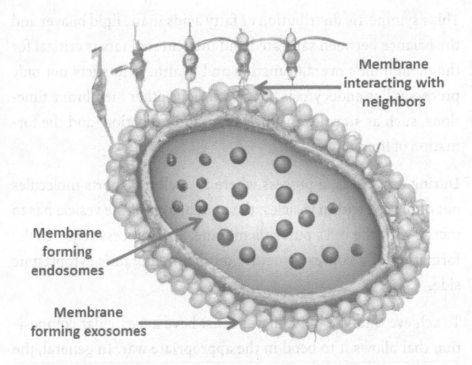

Membrane interacting with neighbors

Membrane forming endosomes

Membrane forming exosomes

Fig. 35: The cell membrane relies on Omega-3 to deliver its messages to the exterior or interior in the form or endo- or exo-somes and to communicate with the neighboring cells and extracellular scaffolding

Is Cholesterol really bad?

Cholesterol makes up a significant portion of blood plasma lipids and because cholesterol can't float freely in the bloodstream, it is transported by lipoproteins such as low-density lipoprotein (LDL) and high-density lipoprotein (HDL). The average cholesterol content of human tissues is indeed roughly 0.5-1% by weight. That is a staggering 1kg on an average 100kg male. The human body needs massive amounts of cholesterol at any given time and just because the LDL particles happen to be found in so called arterial plaques does not establish a causal relationship between cholesterol and heart disease.

Cholesterol is an integral component of all cell membranes and is used in the synthesis of several hormones and bile acids. For that purpose up to 0.2% of the blood can consist of cholesterol by weight.

It is quite surprising how little concrete information we have about such a fundamental aspect of human physiology. However, it's important to note that calculating the exact amount of cholesterol in the human body is complex due to variations in tissue composition and density. The actual amount can vary significantly based on individual factors such as body size, body composition (the proportion of fat to muscle), diet, and genetic predisposition. Also, it's essential to remember that cholesterol isn't uniformly distributed throughout the body; it's concentrated in certain tissues like the brain, liver, and blood.

What we do know is that Cholesterol plays a crucial role in the function and integrity of the cell membrane [100, 101]. Without cholesterol the cell membrane cannot function properly. It cannot maintain nerve function because ion channels cannot open and close properly and neurons cannot exchange vesicles properly. The result is that if the eg. the brain neurons cannot do its job properly and they undergo apoptosis.

In terms of lipid bilayer behavior, cholesterol serves to regulate membrane fluidity. It inserts itself between fatty acid chains, preventing them from packing together and crystallizing, thus maintaining the flexibility of the membrane.

In the context of membrane curvature, which is key for processes such as exocytosis and endocytosis, cholesterol aids by promoting or maintaining the appropriate shape. The molecule's rigid ring structure can influence how lipids pack together and, consequently, the shape of the membrane.

Furthermore, cholesterol too is an essential component of lipid-rafts-microdomains within the cell membrane that serve as organizing centers for the assembly of signaling molecules, influencing membrane fluidity and curvature, and regulating neurotransmission and receptor trafficking.

Our understanding of cholesterol and its role in human health is much more nuanced than the simple good/bad dichotomy often presented. Cholesterol is a complex molecule with multiple functions in the body, and it is not inherently harmful. In fact, it is vital for several key biological processes, including cell membrane structure, hormone production, vitamin D synthesis, and bile production for digestion.

The role of cholesterol, specifically LDL cholesterol, in heart disease is indeed complex and multifaceted. The formation of atherosclerotic plaques, the hallmark of heart disease, involves not just the accumulation of LDL cholesterol in arterial walls, but mainly inflammation and other factors. Inflammation that is largely controlled by a high Omega-6/3 index.

Furthermore, lowering LDL cholesterol levels with statin drugs for over 30 years did not eliminate the risk of heart disease statistically at all. Research even suggests that too low cholesterol levels might be associated with higher mortality, potentially due to the side effects of statins, increased risk of other diseases or health issues [103]. Yi et al 2018 showed in this nature article that a total cholesterol below 140 mg/dl leads up to a 2.5 times higher mortality. "Total Cholesterol levels associated with lowest mortality were

210–249 mg/dL" (which is clearly higher than the recommended maximum of 200 mg/dl). In addition, the whole discussion on "bad cholesterol" that evolved around the so-called "foam cell" and this theory in the development of plaques is now disputed [104, 105]. To add to this discussion it is not the cholesterol that matters but the triglycerides. We know from decades of study there is a linear correlation of Omega-6 and heart disease in the Inuit tribes compared to the US [107]; " attention to cholesterol ignored important evidence that nutritional imbalances in expenditure/intake of energy and in Omega-3/Omega-6 essential fatty acids cause cardiovascular disease:".; "In contrast, concentrations of total cholesterol, LDL cholesterol, and plasma glucose increased as n-3 fatty acid concentrations increased" [106]. "The breakthrough came in the 1970s when Dyerberg and Bang reported that the low incidence of atherosclerotic coronary disease in Greenland Eskimos was due to the high marine lipid content of their diet [108]. It is actually the triglyceride levels that are correlated with cardiovascular disease as discussed in the section on metabolic disease [109].

In conclusion, cholesterol is a vital component of human health, and its role in diseases like heart disease is complex and not fully understood. But it is clear that cholesterol, along with fatty acids like Omega-3 and Omega-6, is vital in ensuring the cell membrane's proper function, which is fundamental to the cell's overall health and functionality. This renders the discussion around "bad cholesterol" futile and coincidental. For a more in-depth discussion around Cholesterol and Triglycerides visit: Omega3health.us/science.

Bonus D

Understanding Statistics and Study biases

Why do some studies show no benefit and why do we often read: "but more research is needed to confirm these findings."?

At this point I feel that it is important to discuss reasons for study biases. There are several reasons why some studies might not show a benefit for a particular intervention, like Omega-3 supplementation, and why researchers often conclude that "more research is needed." Some of the most common issues are:

Lack of Quality Control: Without quality control measures in place, it's hard to ensure that all participants are receiving the same type and quality of supplement. This is especially true for Omega-3 supplements, which can become rancid if not properly stored and handled.

High Dropout Rates: In many studies, a significant proportion of participants discontinue participation before the study is completed. This can bias the results, as the people who drop out might differ in important ways from those who stick with the study.

Subjective Measurements: Diseases like dementia and depression often rely on subjective measures, such as self-reported mood or cognitive function. These measures can be influenced by a host of factors beyond the treatment being studied, making it difficult to isolate the treatment's effects.

Lack of Biomarkers: Without objective biomarkers to measure disease status, it's hard to gauge the true impact of a treatment. This can make the results of a study difficult to interpret and can lead to under- or over-estimation of the treatment's effects.

Short Study Durations: Many studies are only conducted over a short period, such as six months. This might not be enough time to see the full effects of a treatment, particularly for chronic diseases that develop and progress slowly.

Inadequate Control Groups: Without appropriate control groups, it's hard to account for the placebo effect or other factors that might influence the results. For example, people who drop out of a study might have been more likely to experience negative outcomes, which could skew the results if they're not properly accounted for.

Lack of Inflammatory Index Testing: Without testing the inflammatory Omega-6/3 index, it's hard to know how much quality, non-oxidized Omega-3 participants are actually consuming.

All of these issues can contribute to bias in research studies and can make it challenging to draw firm conclusions from the results. That's why researchers often call for more studies to further investigate and confirm their findings. But do more studies really help if they are not done right?

Here is an example of this rancidity problem: Krill oil was shown to be ineffective like in this study [80] where school performance on subject grades or standardized mathematics test scores was tested on subjects taking krill oil for 12 months.

Problem #1: there is no mention of the Omega-6/3 index so we do not know if the krill oil was rancid and if it had any effect on the inflammatory Omega-6 amounts! Krill oil contains up to ⅓ free non-lipid bound Omega-3 which is even more prone to oxidation. The study even states "The krill oil group had a small significant increase in the mean OI3 (Omega-3-index) at all time points. However, very few participants achieved the intended target O3I range of 8-11%."

Problem #2: The study admits that "However, as many participants dropped out and/or were non-adherent, results should be interpreted with caution." Problem #3: 12 months is not enough time to see stem cell changes in the brains of many participants. We know it takes 2-3 years to rectify the enormous deficiency tests in the youth.

In this study on heart failure [91] authors admit: "Ultimately, we suggest that the main failure of Omega-3-PUFAs in clinical trials might be a failure to reach a therapeutically effective concentration."

For more in depth discussions on how study statistics are made go to Omega3health.us/science/#statistics

Problem #3: Understanding statistics can be difficult even to a trained scientist. It is worth mentioning that the odds ratio (OR) can be very misleading: Unlike the HR (hazard ratio) or relative risk (RR) the OR is just a measure relative to the control group (OR = ((1 − p) * RR) / (1 − RR * p). An odds ratio less than 1 indicates a reduction in risk, but it does not directly translate to a percentage decrease in risk. It's a subtle but important distinction in epidemiological studies and one always has to look at the absolute numbers.

What about Krill and Cod liver oil?

In summary, the data presented above clearly indicates that cold water fish like salmon, herring, sardine, and mackerel are the most abundant sources of Omega-3. The iconic Mississippi River, whose image has been featured in this book, is home to several species, including Catfish, Largemouth Bass, and Northern Pike. Although the Omega-3 content in these species is lower, they still provide substantial amounts, approximately 100-200 mg per serving.

As we have mentioned above, most supplements on the market are rancid, Krill oil is no exception. Schuchart et. al. 2011 showed that Krill oil has a significant amount of free DHA and EPA free fatty acid chains which may increase its bioavailibility.

However non-lipid bound DHA is also more prone to oxidation as discussed above[113]. Fish oil in contrast has all of its DHA and EPA bound to lipids. Lipids carrying Omega-3 (particularly phospholipids) are more stable and less subject to oxidation. The fat absorption process is complex and the body takes apart most lipids and triglyceride molecules so PUFAs can be rearranged to the specific needs of the body. They can also be enzymatically converted by desaturase enzymes. This is particularly important to produce eicosanoids.

In summary, there is little data on the bioavailability of PUFAs. The process of cellular functionality and its dependence on Omega-3 PUFAs is very slow and can take years to adjust. As explained above there are many mechanisms for the effects of Omega-3s particularly the Eicosanoid inflammatory cascades. Tests show how your inflammatory index slowly improves over the course of 2-3 years to an optimum below 2:1. In those terms, it would be safer to consume PUFAs in a bound lipid form.

Cod liver oil is known for its high content of vitamins A and D, alongside its Omega-3 fatty acids, EPA (eicosapentaenoic acid), and DHA (docosahexaenoic acid). However, the levels of EPA and DHA can vary depending on the type of fish and their diet.

In cod liver oil, the DHA content tends to be higher than the EPA content. This is mainly due to the fact that DHA is the primary structural component of the brain and retina, and fish like cod have a higher requirement for DHA for maintaining their nervous system, thus resulting in their bodies having a higher concentration of DHA as compared to EPA.

Furthermore, the process of manufacturing cod liver oil may influence the final concentration of these fatty acids. Traditional fermentation processes may preserve more DHA than EPA, whereas modern refining techniques may allow for more controlled levels of both.

Both DHA and EPA are important for human health, and cod liver oil remains a good source of these Omega-3 fatty acids, although the ratio of DHA to EPA may be higher than in other fish oils. However tests show that it is not possible to achieve an Omega-6/3 index below 4:1 with cod liver oil alone.

Finally a disclaimer, all values of Omega-3 and -6 contents in the book vary as is the case for all natural foods. The tables are meant as guidelines and absolute values always need to be verified in laboratory supplement fact analyses. In addition, no medical advice is given herein, nor does this book constitute a replacement for the expertise of a trained medical provider.

Deciding on the best Omega-3 Supplement

Deciding on the oil to consume can often come down to comparing the EPA and DHA contents in each product, particularly in the case of algae-derived vegan oil sources. However, the ultimate determinant of a product's efficacy is the Omega-6/3 index test.

From the insights gained through a million tests performed worldwide, it is currently recommended to use fish oils stabilized with phenolic acid antioxidants. Vitamin E and D are not enough to maintain Omega-3 in an unoxidized state.

An annual Omega-6/3 index test is essential to ensure that the product you are using is functioning correctly. This test should focus on red blood cell (RBC) membranes, not just the liquid part of the blood. A trained nutritionist should interpret the test results.

The daily recommended dosage should be taken with food. A consistent aim should be to bring your Omega-6/3 index below 4:1 within a year and further down to below 2:1 after three years.

How are Omega-3 and Vitamin D connected?

Vitamin D plays a crucial role in several aspects of human health:

- **Bone Health:** Vitamin D helps the body absorb calcium and phosphate from our diet. These minerals are vital for healthy bones, teeth, and muscles.

- **Immune System Function:** Vitamin D plays a significant role in the immune system and can help our bodies fight off bacteria and viruses.

- **Mood and Brain Function:** Some studies have shown a link between vitamin D deficiency and depression. Vitamin D also plays a role in cognitive health, with deficiencies potentially leading to cognitive impairment.

- **Prevention of Chronic Diseases:** Adequate levels of Vitamin D have been associated with a reduced risk for various diseases, including multiple sclerosis and heart disease. There is ongoing research investigating its role in preventing and treating diabetes and cancer.

Omega-3 fatty acids and Vitamin D are both vital nutrients for overall health, but their interplay in the human body is not entirely understood. However, there are several ways in which they appear to be connected:

- **Absorption:** Both Omega-3 fatty acids and Vitamin D are fat-soluble, which means they need fat to be absorbed and stored in the body. This suggests that a diet containing sufficient amounts of healthy fats, including Omega-3s, may aid the absorption of Vitamin D.

- **Immune System Regulation:** Both Omega-3s and Vitamin D play a significant role in immune system regulation. Omega-3s are known for their anti-inflammatory properties, and Vitamin D is crucial for immune response. There is some evidence suggesting that together, they may synergistically boost immune function.

- **Brain Health:** Both nutrients are important for brain health. Omega-3 fatty acids, particularly DHA, are essential for brain function, while Vitamin D is necessary for nerve growth. Low levels of either nutrient have been associated with various neurological conditions.

- **Shared Food Sources:** Fatty fish, one of the best sources of Omega-3 fatty acids, is also one of the few natural dietary sources of Vitamin D. As such, a diet high in fatty fish can be beneficial for both Omega-3 and Vitamin D intake.

- **Impact on Disease Risk:** Emerging research suggests that both Omega-3 and Vitamin D may play a role in reducing the risk of certain diseases, including heart disease and certain types of cancer. Some studies have suggested that the combination of both may have a synergistic effect, potentially offering greater protective benefits.

In summary, while both nutrients have individual roles in the body, their combined impact on health may be significant, and maintaining sufficient levels of both could be beneficial. More research is needed to fully understand their interplay and potential combined effects on health.

This book only contains a subset of the complex topic of Omega-3 science and diseases of fat metabolism.

Tor a deeper look go to omega3health.us/science.

References

[1.] pubmed.ncbi.nlm.nih.gov

[2.] pubmed.ncbi.nlm.nih.gov/?term=omega-3

[3.] pubmed.ncbi.nlm.nih.gov/?term=Simopoulos+ap

[4.] Cordain et. al 2005; pubmed.ncbi.nlm.nih.gov/15699220

[5.] Simopoulos 1999; pubmed.ncbi.nlm.nih.gov/10479232

[6.] N L Selokar 2018; pubmed.ncbi.nlm.nih.gov/30209427

[7.] Rajiv Chowdhury et. al 2012; pubmed.ncbi.nlm.nih.gov/23112118

[8.] Dariush Mozaffarian 2013; pubmed.ncbi.nlm.nih.gov/23546563

[9.] Carol J Fabian 2018; pubmed.ncbi.nlm.nih.gov/29559515/

[10.]Stefania D'Angelo 2020; pubmed.ncbi.nlm.nih.gov/32927614/

[11.] www.seafoodnutrition.org/wp-content/uploads/2018/04/Omega-3-Chart.pdf

[12.] Artemis P Simopoulos 2020; pubmed.ncbi.nlm.nih.gov/21279554/

[13.] www.zinzinotest.com/en/balancetest

[14.] www.zinzinotest.com/en/balancetest?openmap=1#map

[15.] S K Duckett 1993; pubmed.ncbi.nlm.nih.gov/8376232/

[16.] Foods High in Alpha Linolenic Acid (ALA) (myfooddata.com)

[17.] tools.myfooddata.com/nutrient-ranking-tool/Omega-3/Meats/Highest

[18.] Nutrition Facts for Lean Grass Fed Beef Strip Steak (myfooddata.com)

[19.] William S Harris 2004; pubmed.ncbi.nlm.nih.gov/15208005/

[20.] Mihir Parikh 2019; pubmed.ncbi.nlm.nih.gov/31130604/

[21.] Maria Alessandra Gammone 2018; pubmed.ncbi.nlm.nih.gov/30591639/

[22.] Mahsa Jalili 2021; pubmed.ncbi.nlm.nih.gov/33545546/

[23.] Bénédicte Langelier 2010; pubmed.ncbi.nlm.nih.gov/20564231/

[24.] Anamitra Ghosh 2020; pubmed.ncbi.nlm.nih.gov/33298560/

[25.] O Doi, F Doi, F Schroeder, A W Alberts, P R Vagelos 1978; pubmed.ncbi.nlm.nih.gov/656411/

[26.] Ram B Singh 2012; pubmed.ncbi.nlm.nih.gov/22913633/

[27.] wrong Colette M O'Neill 2019; pubmed.ncbi.nlm.nih.gov/27527582/

[28.] Sigrún Huld Jónasdóttir 2019; pubmed.ncbi.nlm.nih.gov/30836652/

[29.] Rosemary J Cater 2021; pubmed.ncbi.nlm.nih.gov/34135507/

[30.] Nicolas G Bazan 2005; pubmed.ncbi.nlm.nih.gov/15912889/

[31.] Anne-Mari Mustonen 2023; pubmed.ncbi.nlm.nih.gov/36768438/

[32.] Ella J Baker 2021; pubmed.ncbi.nlm.nih.gov/33831456/

[33.] Brenda Maddox 2003; pubmed.ncbi.nlm.nih.gov/12540909/

[34.] Alexander V Sorokin 2023; pubmed.ncbi.nlm.nih.gov/37044136/

[35.] Toshinori Hoshi 2013; pubmed.ncbi.nlm.nih.gov/23487785/

[36.] Hidekatsu Yanai 2018; pubmed.ncbi.nlm.nih.gov/29511415/

[37.] Bénédicte Langelier 2020; pubmed.ncbi.nlm.nih.gov/20564231/

[38.]Williams et. al 2006; pubmed.ncbi.nlm.nih.gov/16441943

[39.] Graham C Burdge 2002; pubmed.ncbi.nlm.nih.gov/12323090/

[40.] J B McMillin 1992; pubmed.ncbi.nlm.nih.gov/1332513/

[41.] Clemens von Schacky 2007; pubmed.ncbi.nlm.nih.gov/16979604/

[42.] Dariush Mozaffarian 2004; pubmed.ncbi.nlm.nih.gov/15262826/

[43.] Arzu Ulu 2013; pubmed.ncbi.nlm.nih.gov/23676336/

[44.] Alice V Stanton 2020; pubmed.ncbi.nlm.nih.gov/32963294/

[45.] Bill Lands 2014; pubmed.ncbi.nlm.nih.gov/25373089/

[46.]www.oecd-ilibrary.org/agriculture-and-food/oecd-fao-agricultural-out-look-2015/vegetable-oil-projections-consumption-per-capita-food-use_agr_out-look2015-table132-en

[47.] neurosciencenews.com/omega-3-cognition-aging-21580/

[48.] Carol J Fabian 2018; pubmed.ncbi.nlm.nih.gov/29559515/

[49.] Esha Madan 2022; pubmed.ncbi.nlm.nih.gov/36214625/

[50.] Bethany N Hannafon 2015; pubmed.ncbi.nlm.nih.gov/26178901/

[51.] Anita Vasudevan 2014; pubmed.ncbi.nlm.nih.gov/25193342/

[52.] Alessandra Borsini 2020; pubmed.ncbi.nlm.nih.gov/32636362/

[53.] Marta Crous-Bou 2019; pubmed.ncbi.nlm.nih.gov/31728493/

[54.] Ramin Farzaneh-Far 2010; pubmed.ncbi.nlm.nih.gov/20085953/

[55.] Sawan Ali 2022; pubmed.ncbi.nlm.nih.gov/35189049/

[56.] Janice K Kiecolt-Glaser 2013; pubmed.ncbi.nlm.nih.gov/23010452/

[57.] Alessandra da Silva 2022; pubmed.ncbi.nlm.nih.gov/35661999/

[58.] Danielle Swanson 2012 pubmed.ncbi.nlm.nih.gov/22332096/

[59.] Mohammad Abdur Rashid 2016; pubmed.ncbi.nlm.nih.gov/27651264/

[60.] Jing X Kang 2014; pubmed.ncbi.nlm.nih.gov/24356924/

[61.] Vanessa Danthiir 2011; pubmed.ncbi.nlm.nih.gov/22011460/

[62.] Gordon I Smith 2011; pubmed.ncbi.nlm.nih.gov/21159787/

[63.] Jolan Dupont 2019; pubmed.ncbi.nlm.nih.gov/30784011/

[64.] www.zinzino.com/site/GB/en-gb/blog/health/fish-oil-omega-3-benefits/

[65.] www.zinzino.com/site/GB/en-gb/blog/health/the-omega-3-to-omega-6-ratio/

[66.]portalcris.vdu.lt/server/api/core/bitstreams/acec3865-df77-48c6-849d89a1d2bbdea1/content

[67.] Gao Xin 2021; pubmed.ncbi.nlm.nih.gov/34760272/

[68.] Zhitong Jiang 2022; pubmed.ncbi.nlm.nih.gov/36292774/

[69.] Five Spirits: Alchemical Acupuncture for Psychological and Spiritual Healing; Lorie Dechar

[70.] The Biology of Belief 10th Anniversary Edition: Unleashing the Power of Consciousness, Matter & Miracles; Bruce H. Lipton

[71.]John F Cryan 2019; pubmed.ncbi.nlm.nih.gov/31460832/

[72.] Yimin Han 2022; pubmed.ncbi.nlm.nih.gov/36386584/

[73.] N M Salem 2015; www.ncbi.nlm.nih.gov/pmc/articles/PMC4555191/

[74.] P S Sastry 1985; pubmed.ncbi.nlm.nih.gov/3916238/

[75.] James V Pottala; 2014 pubmed.ncbi.nlm.nih.gov/24453077/

[76.] Lucy M Browning; 2012 pubmed.ncbi.nlm.nih.gov/22932281/

[77.] A F Fotenos 2005; pubmed.ncbi.nlm.nih.gov/15781822/

[78.] Cheng Chen 2020; pubmed.ncbi.nlm.nih.gov/32669395/

[79.] Daniel C Rule 2022; pubmed.ncbi.nlm.nih.gov/36230437/

[80.] Inge S M van der Wurff; 2023 pubmed.ncbi.nlm.nih.gov/36878083/

[81.] Ibrahim M Dighriri 2022; pubmed.ncbi.nlm.nih.gov/36381743/

[82.] Claudia L Satizabal 2022; pubmed.ncbi.nlm.nih.gov/36198518/

[83.] Jane Pei-Chen Chang 2018; pubmed.ncbi.nlm.nih.gov/28741625/

[84.]Janice K Kiecolt-Glaser 2011; pubmed.ncbi.nlm.nih.gov/21784145/

[85.] Mei-Chi Hsu 2020; pubmed.ncbi.nlm.nih.gov/32620164/

[86.] Rossella Avallone 2019; pubmed.ncbi.nlm.nih.gov/31480294/

[87.] Virginia Martín 2010; pubmed.ncbi.nlm.nih.gov/20110596/

[88.]www.nutraingredients.com/Article/2007/11/27/Scientists-connect-DHAto-warding-off-symptoms-of-Parkinson-s

[89.] Simon C Dyall 2015; pubmed.ncbi.nlm.nih.gov/25954194/

[90.] Noemí Fabelo 2011; pubmed.ncbi.nlm.nih.gov/21717034/

[91.] Timothy D O'Connell 2017; pubmed.ncbi.nlm.nih.gov/27986444/

[92.] Rosemary J Cater 2021; pubmed.ncbi.nlm.nih.gov/34135507/

[93.] Ingrid B Helland 2003; pubmed.ncbi.nlm.nih.gov/12509593/

[94.] Sanjay Basak 2021; pubmed.ncbi.nlm.nih.gov/34208549/

[95.] Annelise A Madison 2021; pubmed.ncbi.nlm.nih.gov/33875799/

[96.] H Esterbauer 1993; pubmed.ncbi.nlm.nih.gov/8475896/

[97.] Gerhard Spiteller 2005; pubmed.ncbi.nlm.nih.gov/16270286/

[98.] zinzinowebstorage.blob.core.windows.net/product-sheets/BalanceTest-en-US.pdf

[99.] Rozenn N Lemaitre 2003; pubmed.ncbi.nlm.nih.gov/12540389/

[100.] silvamethod.com/

[101.] Irena Levitan 2010; pubmed.ncbi.nlm.nih.gov/20213557/

[102.] Heike Hering 2003; pubmed.ncbi.nlm.nih.gov/12716933/

[103.] Sang-Wook Yi 2019; pubmed.ncbi.nlm.nih.gov/30733566/

[104.] Sanjay K Singh 2008; pubmed.ncbi.nlm.nih.gov/18293141/

[105.] Valentina Guerrini 2019; pubmed.ncbi.nlm.nih.gov/31732284/

[106.] E Dewailly 2001; pubmed.ncbi.nlm.nih.gov/11566644/

[107.] William E M Lands 2003; pubmed.ncbi.nlm.nih.gov/12848276/

[108.] Arthur A Spector 2019; pubmed.ncbi.nlm.nih.gov/30553403/

[109.] Gregory C Shearer 2012; pubmed.ncbi.nlm.nih.gov/22041134/

[110.] Luc Djoussé 2012; pubmed.ncbi.nlm.nih.gov/22682084/

[111.] H MOHRHAUER 1963; pubmed.ncbi.nlm.nih.gov/14168145/

[112.] Bill Lands 2017; pubmed.ncbi.nlm.nih.gov/28535956/

[113.] J H Song 1997; pubmed.ncbi.nlm.nih.gov/9438988/

[114.] Jan Philipp Schuchardt 2011; pubmed.ncbi.nlm.nih.gov/21854650/

[115.] Meng Yuan 2021; pubmed.ncbi.nlm.nih.gov/33041091/

[116.] H Shimokawa 1998; pubmed.ncbi.nlm.nih.gov/2539756/

[117.] Qianqian Wang 2012; pubmed.ncbi.nlm.nih.gov/22317966/

[118.] Sten Orrenius 2005; pubmed.ncbi.nlm.nih.gov/16408030/

[119.] Valerian E Kagan 2009; pubmed.ncbi.nlm.nih.gov/19285551/

[120.] Matthew L Johnson 2015; pubmed.ncbi.nlm.nih.gov/26010060/

[121.] Cosima Arnold 2010; pubmed.ncbi.nlm.nih.gov/20631419/

[122.] Frank Thielecke 2020; pubmed.ncbi.nlm.nih.gov/33266318/

[123.] Katie M Brown 2019; pubmed.ncbi.nlm.nih.gov/30923750/

[124.] Liana V Basova 2007; pubmed.ncbi.nlm.nih.gov/17319652/

[125.] Marcos Roberto de Oliveira 2017; doi.org/10.1016/j.tifs.2017.06.019

[126.] J B McMillin 1992; pubmed.ncbi.nlm.nih.gov/1332513/

[127.] Chang 2018; pubmed.ncbi.nlm.nih.gov/28741625/

[128.] Dariush Mozaffarian 2004 ; pubmed.ncbi.nlm.nih.gov/15133418/

[129.] Jane Pei-Chen Chang 2018; pubmed.ncbi.nlm.nih.gov/17876193/

[130.] Bill Lands 2016; pubmed.ncbi.nlm.nih.gov/27412006/

[131.] William E M Lands 2003; pubmed.ncbi.nlm.nih.gov/12848276/

[132.] Kylie J Smith 2014; pubmed.ncbi.nlm.nih.gov/24737638/

[133.] Laurie K Mischley 2017; pubmed.ncbi.nlm.nih.gov/29081890/

[134.] Michelle E Fullard 2020; pubmed.ncbi.nlm.nih.gov/32536905/

[135.] Yu-Chia Kao 2020; pubmed.ncbi.nlm.nih.gov/32098382/

[136.] Fernando Gómez-Pinilla 2008; pubmed.ncbi.nlm.nih.gov/18568016/

[137.] Ping-Tao Tseng 2023; pubmed.ncbi.nlm.nih.gov/37150266/

[138.] Mohammad Hassan Sohouli 2023; pubmed.ncbi.nlm.nih.gov/37344075/

[139.] Martin Grootveld 2020; pubmed.ncbi.nlm.nih.gov/32244669/

Please note:

- You can visit the website *pubmed.ncbi.nlm.nih.gov* and enter the PMID number (e.g. /15699220) after *.gov/*.

Acknowledgments

I extend my deepest gratitude to Ingemar Anderson and Kitsap Publishing. Without Ingemar's publishing prowess and unwavering persistence, this book would have remained a dream. I also owe a debt of thanks to ChatGPT, whose assistance in writing and data organization was invaluable. Last but not least, my heartfelt appreciation goes to Birgit Rachold, a fellow practitioner of Chinese Medicine, who introduced me to the remarkable journey of Omega-3. This book is a testament to their collective support and inspiration.

I also want to give thanks to Lukas Richter for help with proofreading and special thanks to Ayver Libes for help with the design of some of the complicated figures.

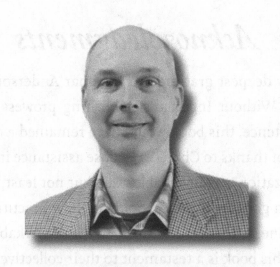

About the Author

Hans-Thomas Richter is the owner of Natureworks Therapeutics in Poulsbo, WA. Hans-Thomas Richter started his studies in Biochemistry at the Medical University of Hannover in 1986. He then went on to a 20-year career in Biomedical Research in Germany and the US and received his Ph.D. in Biochemistry and Biophysics in 1997. Hans-Thomas worked in Academia and Pharmaceutical Industry and has over 20 publications in Medical Research. In recent years he shifted his interests to Natural Medicine, and through his personal success story with Chinese Medicine, he was called to practice Traditional Chinese medicine (TCM). He graduated from the Seattle Institute of Oriental Medicine with a Master in Acupuncture and Oriental Medicine in 2013 and opened a clinic in Poulsbo, WA. Hans-Thomas received his Diplomate of Oriental Medicine and is an East Asian Medical Practitioner certified by the NCCAOM.

His special interests are Internal Medicine with a focus on digestive diseases. In his clinical practice, Hans-Thomas developed treatment programs for several patients with digestive disorders, including IBS, celiac, and ulcerative colitis. Hans-Thomas has experience treating Urogenital diseases such as pelvic inflammations, hemorrhoid bleeding, cystitis, and prostatitis. Hans-Thomas has extensive experience treating musculoskeletal conditions resulting from an overuse injury and trauma and has treated conditions like "frozen" and dislocated shoulders with specialized Tui Na techniques taught in the Zheng Gu tradition by Tom Bisio and Frank Butler. Hans-Thomas has experience rehabilitating fractures using Chinese Medicine techniques, including internal and external Chinese herbs, electro-acupuncture, special Tui Na techniques, Chinese medical cupping, Gua Sha, and Qi Gong. Hans-Thomas also uses Japanese acupuncture and moxibustion techniques when a more gentle approach to healing is required.

Hans-Thomas is also a passionate Golfer and recently treated a legendary leading German senior PGA tour Golfer with an over 50-year history in this sport. It was a pleasure and privilege to help such a distinguished athlete!

Combining Acupuncture, Herbal Medicine, and the intelligent diagnostic approach makes Chinese Medicine outstanding among all other medical treatment modalities known to humankind. The long-term use of Western pharmaceutical drugs often further creates homeostatic imbalances in metabolism. A simple treatment approach to mask the disease symptoms is seldom effective in the long term, and downstream adverse drug effects will further exacerbate the patient's condition and create secondary problems. Hans-Thomas believes that Traditional Chinese Medicine, particularly Chinese Herbal Medicine, can achieve a long-standing homeostatic metabolic balance and thus create a more healthy stage of Yin and Yang, leading to long-lasting health effects.

Hans-Thomas' long-term vision is to combine clinical knowledge of Chinese herbs with modern research further to develop the understanding and application of herbal Medicine. In recent years Research Science has been increasingly investigating the powerful medicinal efficacy of herbal Medicine. Hans-Thomas believes that we need to enter a new era in pharmaceutical and herbal research that incorporates the complex ideas of TCM diagnostics into scientific medical research. We recently added a new natural peptide therapy that regenerates and rejuvenates the body.

Hans-Thomas has also recently published an article on the abuse of sham procedures in the validation of clinical acupuncture outcomes in the International Journal of Complimentary and Alternative Medicine, Acupuncture Studies: *Are They Done with Sham or Scam?*

In addition to his Chinese medical background, Hans-Thomas has been practicing and teaching Yoga and Qi Gong (Chinese breath cultivation) since 1997.

Lastly, some wisdoms

"Don't let your health flounder, take your Omega-3."

"In life, as in the sea, balance is key. Balance your Omega-6 with Omega-3."

"Taking Omega-3 regularly is like keeping your engine well-oiled."

"Don't wait until your health runs aground to start supplementing with Omega-3."

"You wouldn't starve a fish of water, so why starve your body of Omega-3?"

"You can't just float along expecting good health, you have to swim towards it with Omega-3."

"A life without Omega-3 is like a fish without water."

"Dive into better health with Omega-3."

"Just like a fish needs clean water, our bodies need clean sources of Omega-3."

"A little bit of Omega-3 each day keeps inflammation at bay."

"Navigating the sea of life requires the right nutrients—don't forget your Omega-3."

"Like a fish swimming upstream, taking Omega-3 can help you overcome health challenges."

"Omega-3: it's the lifebuoy in the sea of health."